CW01018894

International Perspectives in Geography

AJG Library

Volume 15

Aim and Scope

The AJG Library is published by Springer under the auspices of the Association of Japanese Geographers. This is a scholarly series of international standing. Given the multidisciplinary nature of geography, the objective of the series is to provide an invaluable source of information not only for geographers, but also for students, researchers, teachers, administrators, and professionals outside the discipline. Strong emphasis is placed on the theoretical and empirical understanding of the changing relationships between nature and human activities. The overall aim of the series is to provide readers throughout the world with stimulating and up-to-date scientific outcomes mainly by Japanese and other Asian geographers. Thus, an "Asian" flavor different from the Western way of thinking may be reflected in this series. The AJG Library will be available both in print and online via SpringerLink.

About the AJG

The Association of Japanese Geographers (AJG), founded in 1925, is one of the largest and leading organizations on geographical research in Asia and the Pacific Rim today, with around 3000 members. AJG is devoted to promoting research on various aspects of human and physical geography and contributing to academic development through exchanges of information and knowledge with relevant internal and external academic communities. Members are tackling contemporary issues such as global warming, air/water pollution, natural disasters, rapid urbanization, irregular land-use changes, and regional disparities through comprehensive investigation into the earth and its people. In addition, to make the next generation aware of these academic achievements, the members are engaged in teaching and outreach activities of spreading geographical awareness. With the recent developments and much improved international linkages, AJG launches the publication of the AJG Library series in 2012.

More information about this series at http://www.springer.com/series/10223

Nobuyuki Iwama · Tatsuto Asakawa ·
Koichi Tanaka · Midori Sasaki ·
Nobuhiko Komaki · Masashi Ikeda

Urban Food Deserts in Japan

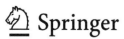 Springer

Nobuyuki Iwama
Ibaraki Christian University
Hitachi, Ibaraki, Japan

Tatsuto Asakawa
Waseda University
Tokorozawa, Saitama, Japan

Koichi Tanaka
Ibaraki University
Mito, Ibaraki, Japan

Midori Sasaki
Hiroshima Shudo University
Hiroshima, Japan

Nobuhiko Komaki
Aichi University
Toyohashi, Aichi, Japan

Masashi Ikeda
Takushoku University
Tokyo, Japan

ISSN 2197-7798   ISSN 2197-7801   (electronic)
International Perspectives in Geography
ISBN 978-981-16-0892-6   ISBN 978-981-16-0893-3   (eBook)
https://doi.org/10.1007/978-981-16-0893-3

This Springer imprint is published by the registered company Springer Nature Singapore Pte Ltd.
The registered company address is: 152 Beach Road, #21-01/04 Gateway East, Singapore 189721, Singapore

Preface

The Purpose of This Book

The purpose of this book is to introduce the Japanese urban food desert (FD) in English. We published a book in Japanese in 2017 (Iwama 2017). The content of this English book is almost the same as the Japanese original. However, we have also added some new information about current Japanese socio-economic environments that strongly connect with FDs.

In Japan, the issue of the worsening living environments of elderly people in poor food-access areas such as rural districts and suburban living complex built in 1960s–70s is drawing attention. These issues are well-known as 'kaimono-nanmin' or 'kaimono jakusya', which in translation means 'disadvantaged shoppers'. We believed that many elderly residents had difficulty shopping in poor food-access areas. Therefore, the Japanese government adopted many countermeasures, such as operating vehicle-based mobile shopping services, shopping bus services, and internet shopping services using mobile terminals (tablets). Local people in many areas also started managing their own support services, such as open-air markets.

However, these services have few users and their business is unprofitable. The managers of these services often say: 'We offer services in poor food-access areas, but few people use our service. Where is "kaimono-nanmin" and "kaimono jakusya"?'.[1] Recently, increasing numbers of people have questioned the existence of 'kaimono-nanmin' and 'kaimono jakusya'. Extensive statistical data certainly suggest that many elderly persons suffer from malnutrition caused by unhealthy eating habits (Ministry of Health, Labour and Welfare 2016). However, few academic studies show clear evidence that the decreased number of nearby grocery shops causes residents' unhealthy eating habits. We have to reconsider elderly people's living environment from an academic perspective.

We are convinced that the most severely impacted living environments are in the central areas of big cities where many elderly people (especially those in single-person households) live and the ties with local communities are very weak. Therefore, in this book, we chose three case study areas—the central area of Tokyo, a prefectural capital city, and a small city (a provincial city)—to clarify the actual state of urban

FD issues through statistical analyses and field surveys. In addition, we discuss countermeasures to FDs (support services for disadvantaged shoppers) that are conducted in many cities. Then, we introduce some remarkable countermeasures.

Definition of the Food Desert Issue

In a broad sense, food deserts (FDs) can be defined as 'the specific areas where many (socially vulnerable) residents' healthy eating habits have deteriorated greatly because of the worsening of their living environments'. Usually, each city has some districts where many of the residents have bad eating habits. Eating habits tend to be worsened by various individual factors, such as food likes and dislikes, unhealthy lifestyle habits, poverty, etc. On the other hand, local factors such as food access and ties with family and neighbours also have a significant influence on residents' eating habits. As regards the former, approaches to each and every person in the form of dietary education and social welfare support are useful. As regards the latter, if we improve the environmental factors (for example, if new shops are opened), residents' eating habits will improve throughout the neighbourhood. FD issues relate to the latter case and it is safe to say that FDs come under geographical and sociological research topics.

We estimate some factors around people's living environment that hinder people's healthy eating habits. In Japan, we generally consider that elderly people's poor eating habits occur due to lowered food access (decrease of nearby grocery shops). It is clear that food access is one of the most important factors in this problem. However, our research points out that decreased social ties with families and local communities (local-level social capital[2]) is also a significant environmental factor that increase elderly people's risk of malnutrition.

Therefore, in this book, we narrowed the definition of current Japanese FDs according to the following two conditions: (1) many socially vulnerable people (especially the elderly) live in a given area, and (2) there is a marked deterioration of shopping environments (a decreasing number of nearby grocery shops and declining food access) and/or the dilution of local ties with families and neighbours (decreased mutual assistance and decline of local social capital).[3]

An Elderly Lady's Eating Habits

We met with Mrs. A in the central area of a prefectural capital city in 2012. She was in her late sixties and lived alone in public housing near the city centre. Her daughter and son-in-law lived in a different prefecture far from her city. Because there were few shops near her house, she always went shopping at a distant supermarket. Through the city council, we requested that she consent to being interviewed/surveyed. She kindly accepted my request and spent about three hours for my interview survey.

She was a good walker and took a walk for about two hours every day. Therefore, her range of activities was very large. She is familiar with this city and informed me clearly about this city's scenic sites and out-of-the-way restaurants. She also told me about her memories of short trips with her old schoolmates and an overseas trip with her daughter and her son-in-law. She had a good geographical sense, so her stories about her trips were very interesting. However, she had moved to this place recently (a few years ago) and knew few of her neighbours. In addition, she did not like neighbourhood communication. She was alone the whole day. She also had problems with her eating habits. Because she was in the workforce for a long time, she did not have much experience of cooking meals. In addition, she did not like fresh vegetables and fish. So, she usually ate ready-to-eat meals and retort or packaged foods. She was concerned about malnutrition. However, few other people worried about her health. We found many elderly people living in similar situations in the area. We were surprised that such areas exist in the centre of big cities.

We often see elderly people walking slowly along lonely shuttered streets to distant supermarkets. Malnutrition caused by the worsening of living environments has increased among elderly people. Eating is a physiological need and a very important part of our lives. We live in a modern and prosperous country where food delivery systems have developed adequately. Therefore, it is safe to say that it is our basic right to get a sufficient quality and quantity of daily food. However, now, when food is plentiful, many people cannot enjoy this basic right. The number of these disadvantaged people is increasing. We can see similar issues in developed countries in Europe and the Americas, such as the UK and the US. In these countries, the main victims of FDs are so-called low-income persons without private cars represented by foreign unskilled labourers living in the inner areas of big cities. European and American FDs are caused by many factors, including the decrease in neighbourhood grocery shops (poor food access), lack of educational opportunities (lack of knowledge about healthy eating), lack of employment opportunities (expansion of poverty, increase of fast food restaurants), etc. In Europe and America, these worsening living environments are related to eating habits and are recognized as social exclusion (socially vulnerable) issues.

Features of FDs differ in Japan when compared with those in Europe/America. Japan is an aging society and FD issues are most serious among the single elderly. In Japan, FD is generally recognized only as a poor food-access issue. The Ministry of Economy, Trade and Industry (METI) defines 'kaimono-jakusya' as an elderly person over 60 years of age who has difficulty in doing daily shopping (METI 2010). The definition of 'kaimono-nanmin' is not clear, but this word usually has the same meaning as 'kaimono-jakusya'. METI estimates that the population of 'kaimono-jakusya' comprises about 6 million people in Japan. On the other hand, the Ministry of Agriculture, Forestry and Fisheries (MAFF) reported more detail and collected research data in 2011. MAFF calculated the number of elderly people over 65 years of age without a car whose house is much more than 500 m from the nearest grocery shop. And they pointed out that the population of 'kaimono-jakusya' is about 3.8 million in Japan. That research considered this issue only as a problem of food access. However, FD is based on social exclusion and the features of Japanese FD must therefore be more diverse in their extent. We must consider the Japanese FD issue from multiple viewpoints.

Disadvantaged Shoppers' Support Services

In Japan, many kinds of disadvantaged shoppers' support services (such as mobile commercial food vans, food and meal delivery services) operate in many poor food-access areas. In particular, mobile food vans have supported many elderly people's daily life. The staff o f hese services are not interested in making a profit for their activities. We are very impressed by their passion to support disadvantaged elderly people.

However, most services do not have enough customers and operate in the red. Many services went bankrupt within a few years of startup. A commercial food van goes around the streets where Mrs. B lives. Although some of her neighbours use this service, she never does. This vehicle also operates in the red. A problem is that these services do not know clearly who needs shopping support, and what kind of support they need. Many staff operate their support services by trial and error and will go bankrupt soon. To consider sustainable and effective countermeasures to tackle FD issues, first we have to consider this issue from an academic viewpoint and clarify who the most serious FD victims are, in what way they suffer from this issue, and where these people live.

Improvements on Our Previous Book

We published our first book 'Japanese food desert issue' in 2011, and newly revised edition in 2013 (Iwama 2011, 2013). In those books, we introduced Japanese food desert studies of the day. At that time, we considered FDs as poor food-access problems (Iwama 2011, 2013). Therefore, in that book, our study focused on poor food-access areas such as those in small cities where shops along central shopping streets had mostly closed down, rural areas where there were few grocery shops, and large-scale housing complexes built in the 1960s on the outskirts of cities, where many residents were over 65 years of age in 2011. We investigated elderly residents' eating habits and shopping behaviours in those areas. As a result, we found that many elderly people did not go shopping frequently and had unhealthy eating habits in local cities and housing complexes. On the other hand, many rural area residents retained good eating habits despite their food access being very poor. Although food access is one of the most important factors of FD, there must also be other factors. In that book, we suggested that ties with neighbours might be another important factor. However, we did not analyse the relationship between social ties and healthy eating habits statistically (not based on evidence).

During the five years since we published our first book, FD studies have developed in Japan. The first development is the advance in social capital (SC) studies. For more detail about SC, please see Chap. 3, Sect. 2. SC refers to ties with family members, friends, neighbours, and so on. If people's SC decreases, their risk of isolation from society becomes higher. As we will mention later, many medical scientists and epidemiologists have pointed out that enriched interactions with friends and families have a good influence on elderly people's health conditions, including depression, self-rated health, nursing care level, and fall incidence rate. SC is generally considered to be an individual factor, but individual forms of SC such as ties with neighbours often accumulate in local areas. Recently, some academic papers have clarified that the quality and quantity of local-level SC are different in each small area such as town streets (For more detail, please see Chap. 3, Sect. 2). And elderly person living in a low-SC area has a higher risk of compromising their health than those in high-SC areas. These research results mean that SC might be an important factor in the occurrence of FDs. If we are isolated from society, it will be difficult to get daily support such as sharing meals with neighbours. These supports are essential for elderly people to maintain healthy eating habits. In addition, the isolation might deprive people of their will to live and may reduce health awareness.

The second development is the interest in urban FDs. As Chaps. 4–6 show, large-scale FDs exist in big cities such as Tokyo and prefectural capital cities. Moreover, the population of elderly residents keeps increasing rapidly in urban areas. This fact means that FDs will expand more in big cities in the near future. To protect elderly people's living environments, we have to analyse the occurrence factors of urban FDs and clarify correctly where the FDs actually exist.

The third development is quantitative and empirical research using large-scale data. Recently, socio-economic research using big data has shown good progress. Governments also support this research and they are building platforms for big data databases with protection for personal information. So, it is becoming more convenient for us to use these big data for academic research. Actually, measuring food access has becoming easier because of big data. Although measuring SC is still difficult, it will be easier in the near future.

This book is the sequel to our previous book and introduces our new FD studies undertaken since 2011. The features of this book are as follows:

(1) Redefinition of Japanese FD issues from the viewpoints of food access and SC.
(2) Empirical research in central areas of big cities (central Tokyo, prefectural capital city, and local city).
(3) Understanding of actual conditions underlying Japanese FDs and factor analysis (development of new FD maps based on food access and SC).
(4) Introduction of remarkable measures to combat FD issues.

Development of New FD Maps

One of the main subjects of this book is answering the question, 'where are the FDs located?'. I think many would ask the same question. If we have accurate FD maps, we can offer suitable support services to the people who really need help. Geographers have a responsibility to make these maps correctly. This is a very heavy and difficult responsibility. Many kinds of living-environment factors relate to the elderly people's unhealthy eating habits (not only individual attributes such as poverty, solitude, and decreased strength, but also local factors including food access and SC). FD maps must include these factors.

The FD studies so far have been based on the blank areas of maps of grocery shop locations (so-called food-access maps). In our previous book, we called these maps 'Food desert maps'. However, as we will mention later, there is not always an overlap of the location of poor food-access areas and the distribution of elderly people with poor eating habits (Chaps. 4–6). To understand FD issues correctly, we have to reconsider both food access and SC.

We can measure food access relatively easily. But there is no established statistical database about SC (individual data which show the ties with family members and neighbours), and to measure local-level SC by ourselves, we would have to conduct a large-scale questionnaire survey of all elderly residents within the research areas. To do this survey, full support of governments and self-government associations is necessary. In addition, significant funding is required to carry out the questionnaire survey.

In Chap. 3, we show two maps illustrating the distributions of disadvantaged shoppers in Tokyo 23 Wards and Minato Ward. Minato Ward is one of the richest areas in Tokyo 23 Wards. These maps are made using demand and supply balance data on residents and shops. In this chapter, we also describe how to make several types of food access maps. In Chap. 5, we show a new FD map created using two indexes: food access and SC. This map is revolutionary. However, we made this new map only in one city because of the difficulty of collecting each resident's data about SC.

The Structure of This Book

The structure of this book is as follows. In Chap. 1, we outline FD issues. In particular, first, we discuss previous overseas studies. Then, we introduce recent Japanese FD studies and definitions o f Japanese FDs.

In Chap. 2, we introduce problems associated with Japan's aging society and analyse elderly people's living environments using statistical data. In particular, we focus on the living environments within big cities.

In Chap. 3, we consider two important factors: food access and SC. With regard to food access, we introduce recent research trends and show some ways of making food access maps. With regard to SC, we introduce recent research trends and show two types of measurement procedures of SC.

In Chap. 4, we consider the existence of FD and its features in central Tokyo, where the case study area is Minato Ward. Minato Ward has a complex population composition. Although Minato Ward is one of the richest areas in Japan, the problem of poverty is also remarkable there. Meiji-Gakuin University has researched the poverty problem in this area. In addition, we analysed the main factors of elderly residents' bad eating habits from two viewpoints: individual factors (age, gender, financial condition, etc.) and living environment (food access and SC). In this book, we introduce an outline of above research.

In Chap. 5, we introduce our research about the case study of a prefectural capital city located on the outskirts of the Tokyo metropolitan area. First, we clarify the distribution of elderly people with a high risk of malnutrition. Second, we look for main factors that seriously decrease elderly people's healthy eating habits using multilevel analyses. Third, we extract FDs and clarify their features.

In Chap. 6, we describe our study in a local city located on the outskirts of the Tokyo metropolitan area. This city has two different types of areas: a commuter town of Tokyo and a traditional agricultural area. In this chapter, we clarify the distribution of elderly people with a high risk of malnutrition and analyse main factors associated with elderly residents' unhealthy eating habits. In this chapter, we also consider the effectiveness of the support services for disadvantaged shoppers. A mobile food van service operates in this city. So, we make a comparison between the services offered and the actual conditions of FDs in the city. Then we suggest the advantages and disadvantages of this service, and point out some improvement plans.

In Chap. 7, we introduce some remarkable countermeasures (support services) to combat FDs in Japan and consider key ways of solving this issue. Typical countermeasures are mobile food vans, and food and meal delivery services. There are many kinds of services available. Their operating bodies are also diverse, including the Japanese government, local governments, private companies, and local residents. Unfortunately, almost all of these services are unprofitable. On the other hand, some people are trying to restructure their services effectively to secure their profitability. In this chapter, we organize Japanese countermeasures for FDs in systematic order and introduce some remarkable case examples.

Notes

1. METI reported 62.3% of businesses that operate support services for elderly people answered, 'I think disadvantaged shoppers must exist. But I do not know where they live'. http://www.meti.go.jp/policy/economy/distribution/kai monoshien2010.htm (Japanese). Accepted 13 February 2020.
2. Social capital refers to social networks (ties with people and groups) and normative consciousness based on trust and reciprocity. More detail, please see Chap. 3 sect. 2.
3. In our previous book (Iwama 2011), we defined the food desert issue as 'socially vulnerable groups' health problems that often occur in places that meet the

following two conditions: (1) fresh food supply system is broken, and (2) many socially vulnerable groups reside here' (p1). In this definition, we defined condition (1) based on the following two factors: spatial factor (the extent of the physical distance between the residence and the nearest grocery shop) and social factor (the extent of the economic and mental distance caused by poverty and social isolation). However, we have not paid enough attention to the social factor. Therefore, in this book, we redefine Japanese FD issues from the viewpoints of food access and social capital.

Hitachi, Japan	Nobuyuki Iwama
Tokorozawa, Japan	Tatsuto Asakawa
Mito, Japan	Koichi Tanaka
Hiroshima, Japan	Midori Sasaki
Toyohashi, Japan	Nobuhiko Komaki
Tokyo, Japan	Masashi Ikeda

References

Iwama N (ed) (2011) Food deserts issues: food deserts and isolated society. Association of Agriculture and Forestry Statistics, Tokyo (Japanese)

Iwama N (ed) (2013) Newly-revised edition: food deserts issues: food deserts and isolated society. Association of Agriculture and Forestry Statistics, Tokyo (Japanese)

Iwama N (ed) (2017) Urban food deserts issues: urban food deserts in low-social capital areas. Association of Agriculture and Forestry Statistics, Tokyo (Japanese)

Ministry of Economy, Trade and Industry (2010) Research report of distribution system which supports local life infrastructure (Japanese). http://www.meti.go.jp/report/downloadfiles/g10 0514a03j.pdf (Japanese). Accessed 14 Aug 2020

Ministry of Health, Labour and Welfare (2016) National health and nutrition surveys in 2018 (Japanese). https://www.mhlw.go.jp/stf/newpage_08789.html (Japanese). Accessed 14 Aug 2020

Contents

About the Authors

Nobuyuki Iwama

- Unified the complete work, responsible for analysis from a urban geographical viewpoint.
- Professor of Ibaraki Christian University, Department of Literature.
- Chief Literary Works:

  Iwama N (ed) (2011) Food deserts issues: food deserts and isolated society. Association of Agriculture and Forestry Statistics, Tokyo. (Japanese)

  Iwama N (ed) (2013) Newly revised edition: food deserts issues: food deserts and isolated society. Association of Agriculture and Forestry Statistics, Tokyo. (Japanese)

  Iwama N (ed) (2017) Urban food deserts issues: urban food deserts in low-social capital areas. Association of Agriculture and Forestry Statistics, Tokyo. (Japanese)

Tatsuto Asakawa

- Responsible for analysis from a urban sociological viewpoint.
- Professor of Waseda University, School of Human Sciences.
- Chief Literary Works:

  Kurasawa S and Asakawa T (ed) (2004) Newly revised edition: social map of Tokyo metropolitan area 1975–1990. Sanbi Printing Co., Ltd, Tokyo. (Japanese)

  Asakawa T (2016) Changes in the socio-spatial structure in the Tokyo metropolitan area: social area analysis of changes from 1990 to 2010, Development and Society 45(3):537–562. (English)

  Asakawa T and Hashimoto K (2020) Social polarization and urban space: social map of Tokyo metropolitan area 1990–2010. Kajima Institute Publishing Co., Ltd., Tokyo. (Japanese)

Koichi Tanaka

- Responsible for spatial analysis using Geographic Information System (GIS).
- Professor of Ibaraki University, College of Humanities and Social Sciences.
- Chief Literary Works:

Araki H, Tanaka K, et al. (2016) Delivering relief supplies: geography's contribution to reducing secondary damage from widespread disasters. E-Journal GEO 11(2):526–551. (Japanese with English abstract)

Tanaka K, Komaki N, and Kainuma E (2016) Accessibility evaluation of evacuation from tsunami on the basis of geographical condition: a case study of coastal area in Tokushima prefecture. Theory and Application of GIS 24(2):97–103. (Japanese with English abstract)

Tanaka K (2014) Transport geography in Japan. Journal of Transport Geography 34:305–306. (English)

Midori Sasaki

- Responsible for analysis of local community.
- Professor of Hiroshima Shudo University, The Faculty of Human Environmental Studies.
- Chief Literary Works:

Sasaki M, et al. (2018) Rice Industry Trends in Australia. Geographical Space 11(1):63–77. (Japanese with English abstract)

Hiroshima Sudo University Forest Biomass Research Group (2013) Regional Development Using Forest Biomass. Chuokeizai-Sha, Inc., Tokyo. (Japanese)

Sasaki M and Ishikawa T (2012) Promotion of research towards low-carbon societies: contributions of the international research network for low-carbon societies. Environmental Research Quarterly 165:176–183. (Japanese with English abstract)

Nobuhiko Komaki

- Responsible for creating food access maps.
- Professor of Aichi University, Faculty of Regional Policy.
- Chief Literary Works:

Ito S, Arima T, Komaki N, Hayashi T, and Suzuki K (ed) (2012) Towards a practical geography. Kokon Shoin, Tokyo.

Komaki N (2018) Conditions of commercial accumulation in city centres resulting from authorized central district revitalization basic plans by industry composition. E-journal GEO 13(1):127–139. (Japanese with English abstract)

Komaki N (2016) A development of community movement in downtown toyohashi city: a case study of 'the urban art event "Sebone"' in Toyohashi City. Aichi University Journal of Regional Policy Studies 5(2):19–35. (Japanese with English abstract)

Masashi Ikeda

- Responsible for developing systems.
- Professor of Takushoku University, Faculty of Commerce.
- Chief Literary Works:

Ikeda M (2020) A study of the distribution characteristics of cut vegetables. Takushoku University Research in Management and Accounting 117:59–73. (Japanese)

Ikeda M (2018) Construction of the annual procurement system and the significance of the corporate entrance into agriculture by a restaurant chain: a case study of MOS food services, Inc. Takushoku University Research in Management and Accounting 112:207–225. (Japanese)

Ikeda M (2010) A Study of the Supply-Demand Adjustment System: Case Study of Pal System. Takushoku University Research in Management and Accounting 89:145–163. (Japanese)

Chapter 1
The Definition of Japanese Food Desert Issues

Abstract In this chapter, we introduce Japanese food desert (FD) issues and their socioeconomic backgrounds. In a broad sense, FDs can be defined as 'specific areas where many (socially vulnerable) residents' healthy eating habits have deteriorated greatly because of the declining quality of living environments (local factors).' However, for a strict definition of FDs, we must consider living environments carefully. We have researched many locations, such as central Tokyo, other large cities, dormitory suburbs, smaller cities, remote agricultural and mountainous areas, and disaster-stricken areas. Then, we narrowed the current definition of Japanese FDs according to the following two conditions: (1) many socially vulnerable people (especially the elderly) live there and (2) there is a marked deterioration of shopping environments (a decreasing number of nearby grocery stores and declining food access) and/or the dilution of local ties with families and neighbors (decreased mutual assistance and decline of local social capital).

Keywords Definition of Japanese food desert issues · Socially vulnerable people · Poor food access · Dilution of local ties with families and neighbors

1.1 What Are Food Desert Issues?

1.1.1 Isolated Elderly People Who Live in Big Cities

Mr. B drew my attention to the issue of Japanese urban food deserts (FDs). We met him in 2012. He was over 80 years old, and he lived in the center of a prefectural capital city with his wife. A staff member at the city office of the senior citizens' welfare division invited him to talk to us and gave us his address in the center of the downtown district. It was not our home city, but we were familiar with it. Although we did not believe there were any private homes in the area, we arrived at the address 30 min before the appointment. The address was in a backstreet to the main shopping street. There were many fashionable bars and miscellaneous goods shops, as well as fountain and water features. here were many seats and a large clock tower. This area appeared to be under redevelopment by the government. The backstreet was very busy at night with young office workers. As expected, we could not find any private houses there. We asked some clerks from the nearby miscellaneous goods shops, but no one knew his address. We were in trouble and we called him directly by phone. He soon answered and kindly gave us directions. He told us, 'I am sorry, but I have serious back pain and I cannot pick you up. Please look behind the clock tower and you will find our house's entrance soon.' Therefore, we looked behind the tower and found a small door with his nameplate in the hedge. Although Mr. B is an elderly man aged over 80 years, he was energetic and quiet. During the survey interview, we found him clever and erudite. We admired and respected him. His house is located in a bustling street mainly composed of fashionable pubs and miscellaneous goods shops. However, this street used to be a typical shopping street comprising many kinds of stores selling goods such as groceries, commodities, and clothing. He had managed a stationery store with his wife for a long time. This store was next to his house, and it had been a long-established shop that had lasted for three generations. His wife was a good partner and she managed the business in general, performing tasks such as waiting on customers and stocking up on stationery. They were extremely busy when running the business and had no time to cook for themselves. Therefore, they usually bought ready-cooked meals/dishes at neighboring food stores and ate them with their family. Now, they have closed their stationery store and let the property to a tenant. The couple have two daughters. The elder daughter lives in Tokyo and the younger one lives in a suburb of this city.

Mr. B was very busy caring for his wife, who suffers from dementia. Until 2007, he and his wife went to a nearby welfare center for the elderly and enjoyed chatting and singing karaoke with their friends. Because of the worsening of his wife's symptoms, they had to stop going to the welfare center. Although she suffers from dementia, Mrs. B has sufficient stamina to go outside and often wanders. Sometimes, she is found by the police in faraway cities and Mr. B goes to pick her up by taxi. Once, she was even mistakenly arrested by the police for shoplifting in a large store. For patients with dementia, nursing home fees are higher than for others. In addition, few nursing homes accept them, so he had no choice but to care for his wife by himself. The only time he can relax is just half a day per week when his wife goes for a short stay at the day care center for seniors. He kindly sacrificed his important leisure time for us and talked about their living environment for three hours. We really appreciated his kindness. He told us, 'I understand that nursing homes are too busy to care for dementia patients like my wife. However, our society should understand our tough living environment better.'

There used to be many independent stores along this street, and their owners and their families lived in the district. They maintained good relationships in this community and established their own local association. However, after the deregulation of large stores in the 1990s (for details, please see Chapter 1, Sect. 1.2.3), independent stores disappeared one after another, and chain establishments, such as pubs and convenience stores, have been established in the shopping streets. Mr. B's street has also changed dramatically. The clerks at the chain stores usually live in suburban residential districts and commute to the stores from their houses every day. The local population has rapidly decreased. Now, few elderly families like that of Mr. B and his wife live in this area. Their local association has dissolved, and he has not met his neighbors for a long time.

Mr. B has trouble with his back and must care for his wife throughout the day, so he has too little time and mental stamina to go shopping and cook by himself. His daughters live far from this city and it is difficult for them to take care of their parents. In addition, Mr. B and his wife's ties with their neighbors are very weak. He has few friends and relatives on whom he can rely in times of trouble. He uses a private food distribution service on weekdays. The meals are too large for him, so he shares them with his wife. There is no service on weekends, so he usually buys bread and lunch from nearby convenience stores. He is very concerned about his own and his wife's eating habits, but he has no other choice.

After the study of FD issues in this city, we held a briefing session for the office staff of the prefectural government office and city hall. In this session, I mentioned that many elderly people with poor eating habits, such as Mr. B, live in the city center. Then, one officer asked us, 'The city center is an upper-class residential area. Do such elderly people really live there?' I was very surprised that some local officers did not recognize the seriously deprived living environment of the elderly residents of the city center. Certainly, there are many shoppers and lively cityscapes in the center. The current trend of people returning to the city center has caused the number of high-rise apartments to increase. Many of their residents are relatively young and rich. The officer had good reason to believe that FD issues do not arise in the city center. However, in apartments above chain stores and in the back streets, many people such as Mr. B live in the shadows and need support. In addition, less noticeably, many low-income people live in decrepit houses left behind after urban development. Many of these people are elderly. With a declining birth rate and an aging population, it is estimated that the number of elderly people will increase further in urban areas such as Tokyo. The encounter with Mr. B became an important turning point for our study of FDs in Japan.

1.1.2 The Definition of 'Food Deserts'

Almost all cities have areas where concentrations of people with unhealthy eating habits live. An internist from a regional hospital told us in 2012, 'I can't show you the patients' charts. But it seems that the residential districts of the patients with diseases associated with diet, such as kidney disease and obesity, are concentrated in specific areas.' This means that elderly people's eating habits may be affected by geographic factors. Eating habits certainly deteriorate because of individual attributes or factors such as food preferences, irregular lifestyles, or economic conditions (e.g., Yagi et al. 2019). On the other hand, living environments (local factors), such as districts where there have been decreases in the number of nearby grocery stores, also have a severe impact on daily eating habits. In the former case, promoting social welfare services, such as nutritional education, is important for improving eating habits. In the latter case, if we alleviate geographical and spatial problems, the eating habits of residents will improve at the regional level.

In a broad sense, FDs can be defined as 'the specific areas where many (socially vulnerable) residents' healthy eating habits have deteriorated greatly because of the worsening of their living environments (local factors).' However, to define FDs more strictly, we must consider living environments more carefully. Current FD studies tend to focus only on food access (the declining number of nearby grocery stores) (e.g., Yakushiji 2015; Ohashi et al. 2017; Kikushima and Takahashi 2018). However, the FD issue is not simple. It is a highly complex social problem based on social exclusion. There are many local factors that may have negative influences on residents' eating habits. The most influential local factor may be different in each area, region, and country.

We have researched many places, such as central Tokyo, other large cities, dormitory suburbs, smaller cities, remote agricultural and mountainous areas, and disaster-stricken areas (Iwama 2011, 2013). The most serious victims of Japanese FDs are elderly people isolated from their families and neighbors. If they are isolated from society, it becomes very difficult to obtain support for tasks such as shopping, sharing food and meals, dining with families and neighbors, receiving advice on healthy eating habits, and so on. Intellectual activities are essential to maintain independence and an intellectual life; for example, exploration, creative pursuits, and leisure activities. Isolation often drains the energy that elderly people require to live and impedes the intellectual activities that are important to maintain independent lives (Kumagai 2011). The residents' eating habits easily deteriorate where ties with families and neighbors are weak, even where there is adequate access to food. These areas constitute FDs. On the other hand, in some areas with poor food access, residents procure food through bulk purchases by private car, sharing food and meals with neighbors and receiving support from children who live nearby. These do not constitute FDs.

From these points, we narrowed the definition of current Japanese FDs according to the following two conditions: (1) many socially vulnerable people (especially the elderly) live there and (2) there is a marked deterioration of shopping environments (fewer nearby grocery stores and declining food access) and/or the dilution of local ties with families and neighbors (decreased mutual assistance and decline of local social capital[1]).

1.2   The Structure of Food Deserts

1.2.1   Declining Nutrition of Elderly Residents

Although we are living in what is called a 'satiation period', a form of malnutrition is spreading among elderly people in Japan. However, it is often difficult for young people to notice the existence of elderly people with shopping disadvantages and poor eating habits. The weakening of connections within local communities also hides the existence of these elderly people. Fortunately, some recent media broadcasts have reported this issue in Japan and FD issues are generally recognized by many people. However, FDs are invisible and sometimes misunderstood. Many people blame large retail companies and the government for emptying traditional shopping streets and expanding FDs. However, FDs are a structural problem stemming from many factors related to the aging population and changes in lifestyle. Therefore, I am sure that the FD issue is not the fault of specific companies or the government.

Figure 1.1 shows the relationship between FDs and elderly people's poor eating habits. This model is based on past research (Iwama 2011, 2013). Socially vulnerable people, such as the elderly and the poor, have always existed. So far, environments with minimum living standards, such as easy access to grocery stores and hospitals, have been maintained by the government. Moreover, families and neighbors have protected elderly people. Therefore, the socially vulnerable can maintain a certain quality of life. However, many elderly people's eating habits have recently deteriorated dramatically. Poor eating habits directly increase the risk of malnutrition. Individual and local factors have contributed to this problem. Individual factors are

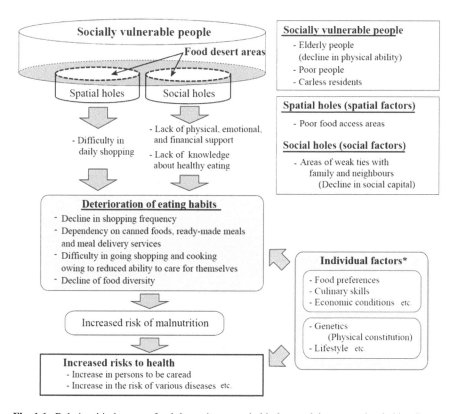

Fig. 1.1 Relationship between food desert issues and elderly people's poor eating habits. *Source* Iwama ed. (2017). *Note* Individual factors are personal attributes and circumstances. However, social factors also influence individual factors (Kondo 2007)

based on personal circumstances, such as food preferences, culinary skills, economic conditions, genetics (constitution), and lifestyle.[2] On the other hand, FD issues are mainly related to local factors, such as food access and social capital, which are based on living environments. Poor eating habits cause many illnesses, such as diabetes and kidney failure, that pose long-term care risks for elderly people.

Recently, large spatial holes (geographical areas with poor food access) and social holes (areas of weak ties with family and neighbors) have appeared in many places such as large cities, aging housing districts, agricultural villages, mountain villages, and fishing villages (Iwama 2011, 2013). If an elderly person lives in a spatial hole, owing to poor food access, they have serious difficulty going shopping. If they are in a social hole, owing to weak social capital, they have serious difficulty in obtaining various kinds of support (shopping assistance, sharing food and meals, dining together, etc.) from their families or neighbors. Poor social capital also causes isolation from society. These holes in the living areas of socially vulnerable people can be defined as FDs.

An elderly person in one of these holes often has problems such as decreased shopping frequency and excessive dependency on canned foods, ready-made meals, and meal delivery services. To maintain self-sufficiency and independence, shopping, cooking, and dining with others are very important activities, as many academic studies have shown (Kumagai 2011). Recently, some companies have started ready-made meal delivery services. However, to maintain their independence, elderly people should not depend entirely on these convenient services. As a result of these problems, their diets are very unbalanced, and the risk of malnutrition is greater. Decreased intellectual activity and the loss of reasons to live also impair eating habits. The deterioration of eating habits is strongly influenced by individual attributes. In addition, genetics (physical constitution) and lifestyle (rhythm of life, drinking or smoking) have a significant impact on eating habits. However, as mentioned above, living environment (geographical) factors are also important in this regard. FDs are very much a local geographical matter. Therefore, a geographical perspective is vital to understand this social issue.

1.2.2 The Increasing Number of Socially Vulnerable People

Socially vulnerable people have always existed, so why has the FD issue emerged only recently? The increase in the number of socially vulnerable people is strongly connected to the aging population. The aging of Japanese society is well known. The population of people over 65 years old is 35.6 million, and 28.1% of the population were elderly in 2018 (Ministry of Internal Affairs and Communications 2019). The proportion of elderly people will increase rapidly in urban areas such as the Tokyo, Osaka, and Nagoya metropolitan areas (Japanese Cabinet 2015a). Those born between 1925 and 1950 are the so-called 'generation of the population transition period' (for details, please see Chapter 2). They are the first generation who were born to and grew up in large families but had small families of their own (nuclear families). The elderly now are from this generation; they are the first generation to suffer from weak ties with families (and lack family support). Recently, welfare budgets for the elderly have been reduced. Therefore, poverty is serious for some low-income single-person and couple households (with no support from their children). These people are the most socially vulnerable people in modern Japan and the most serious victims of Japanese FDs.

1.2.3 The Expansion of Spatial Holes (Spatial Factors)

We argue that current changes in trading and shopping environments are the main reason for the expansion of spatial holes. Trading and shopping environments are changing rapidly, owing to changes in urban construction and the dramatic reorganization of logistical systems (Arai and Hashimoto 2004). The deregulation of large retailers has an especially strong influence on this dramatic reorganization of logistical systems. The *Large-Scale Retail Store Law* adopted in 1974 has strictly controlled large-scale retailers and protected small retailers' activities. In fact, this act protected small retailers, such as independent stores and those in central shopping streets, for many decades.

However, the government weakened the act gradually during the 1990s and completely repealed it in 2000. This policy shift was caused by (1) external pressure from the US (which wanted to enter the Japanese market in the 1980s) and (2) the government view that small retailers were over-protected, reducing large retailers' competitiveness as a result. Currently, the Japanese government administers the industry through three acts: the *Large-Scale Retail Store Location Act*, the *City Planning Act* (revised in 2006), and the *Central City Invigoration Act*. These three acts are called 'the three town development laws.' The *Large-Scale Retail Store Location Act* is intended to protect the living environment and is lenient to large retailers. Land use restrictions are not strict in suburbs. Therefore, since the 1990s, this restriction has accelerated the relocation of large retailers to suburbs. As a result, the recent hollowing out of central shopping streets in Japan has been remarkable (especially in smaller cities).

Recent social systems have sought economic rationality. They have also created spatial holes. Many retail companies and public transportation companies, such as bus companies, do not like to operate in rural or remote areas. They withdraw from areas with low population density and thus expand areas with poor food, poor medical services, and poor transportation. For public buses, the revision of the government subsidy system in 2001 and the deregulation of bus services had a severe impact on the public bus system. Owing to these changes, many different businesses have entered the public bus industry, generating strong competition between newcomers and existing bus companies. The government has reduced the subsidy. As a result, many companies have reduced their operations in unprofitable less-populated areas, such as remote islands and rural areas. Some of these areas cannot afford to offer alternatives to carless residents. We must consider which forms of public transportation should be made available in unprofitable areas.

To reduce the hollowing out of central shopping streets, the Japanese government has considered a 'compact city policy' since the early 2000s. A compact city is a sustainable city where (1) urban facilities such as shopping streets, hospitals, and housing have been arranged optimally in city centers, and phenomena such as the hollowing out of central urban districts are not seen (there is urban revitalization and sustainable economic development). (2) Residents do not rely on private cars, and all kinds of urban facilities are within walking distance (reducing environmental burdens caused by transportation). (3) Poorly planned developments in suburban districts are strongly restricted (to prevent suburban sprawl and conserves the environment) (EC-Environment 1990; Kaido 2001). The *City Planning Act* was revised in 2006. This revised act promotes the compact city policy and has partly restricted the opening of large stores in suburban districts. In addition, the government established the *Local Shopping Mall Revitalization Act* in 2009 to support approved shopping district revitalization projects by local shopping center promotion associations. The government has also discussed the improvement of public transportation systems using light rail transit (LRT) systems. Since 2000, many high-rise apartments have been built in city centers and population redistribution to the city centers has increased in many large and small cities.

Several cities demonstrate the results of the compact city policy. For example, Aomori city, the provincial capital of Aomori prefecture, has promoted the new policy. This policy separates Aomori city into three zones: the inner areas (the central districts), the middle areas (suburbs), and the outer areas (rural and agricultural areas). The city government promotes different land uses and public transportation policies in each zone based on its characteristics and attempts to suppress urban sprawl. Toyama city, the capital of Toyama prefecture, has tried to rebuild a walkable community using LRT and public bus networks. However, these cities' projects encounter many difficulties.[3]

So far, the compact city policy has not been successful in Japan. Many people still travel to large shopping malls in private cars, and almost all cities except for a few large ones have a serious hollowing out of central shopping streets.

1.2.4 The Expansion of Social Holes (Social Factors)

The family structure in Japan has changed since around 1990. This is one of the main reasons for the expansion of social holes. For about 60 years after World War 2, the family structure in Japan changed as follows. The country emerged from poverty (1945–early 1970s), achieved a reasonable standard of living (the later 1970s–1980s), and entered an age of diversification (1990s–the present) (Hirayama 2006). In the past, on the way to achieving a reasonable standard of living, everyone aimed to 'get a job,' 'get married,' and 'have babies' as a matter of course. However, these are no longer common life goals. Because of the diversity of life, some people do not pursue jobs, marriage, or babies. Current social issues, such as rising unemployment, widening disparities, and uncertainty about the future, have also accelerated changes in life goals. These changes in goals weaken ties with families and may cause the decay of the usual family support systems.

The rarefaction of local communities is also a major reason for the expansion of social holes. Japanese Cabinet Office pointed out that 52.8% of survey respondents answered 'we maintain good relationships with neighbors' in 1975. However, this score had decreased to 10.7% by 2007 (Japanese Cabinet 2007). There are many factors that weaken the ties of local communities; for example, changing attitudes toward the community (an increase in the number of people who do not appreciate extensive communications with neighbors), more newcomers (whose workplaces are far from their residences; they commute for long distances every day and do not become involved in the local community), the increasing number of single-person households (nuclearization of the family, increased numbers of unmarried people), changes in living environments (increased proportions of rental apartments and rapid turnover of the residents), and so on. In fact, many people do not like close communications among neighbors (close relationships are common in rural agricultural areas. There, people help each other. However, sometimes neighbors violate residents' privacy) (Japanese Cabinet 2015b). On the other hand, many people want to moderate their relationships with neighbors (they want to maintain their privacy but need help from neighbors when they are in difficulty). Moreover, many people want to contribute to the local community by participating in social activities such as the work of nonprofit organizations and volunteer associations. These tendencies became popular after the Han-Shin Awaji Earthquake disaster in 1995. However, many people are too busy to participate in these activities.

The weak ties with families and neighbors (so-called low-level social capital) might expand social holes and deteriorate the living environments of the socially vulnerable people.

1.2.5 Regional Differences in the Main Causes of FD Issues

Figure 1.2 shows regional differences in the main factors that deteriorate residents' healthy eating habits (Iwama 2011, 2013). In rural areas, such as depopulated agricultural, mountain, and fishing districts, there is a lack of grocery stores. Poor food access is the primary reason for the expansion of FDs in these areas. On the other hand, residents generally maintain strong ties with families and neighbors in these areas. Therefore, neighbors usually help disadvantaged elderly shoppers and thus maintain their living environment. However, more recently, many people from the younger generation have taken jobs in big cities and have moved from rural areas. Therefore, we are concerned that elderly people's living environments may become worse in the near future.

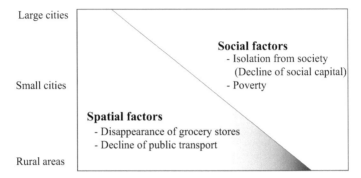

Fig. 1.2 Regional differences in main factors that deteriorate residents' healthy eating habits. *Source* Iwama ed. (2011)

In small provincial cities, both spatial and social factors influence FD issues. Because of the hollowing out of central shopping streets, there are many areas with poor food access. In some areas of small cities, residents maintain close local communities. However, in other areas, such as downtown districts, local communities have already been weakened. In these poor community areas, many elderly people are isolated from society.

In large cities, such as central Tokyo, social factors have a significant influence on residents' eating habits. Although food access in these areas is relatively good, weak ties in the local community and families are very serious. Isolated elderly people usually do not find life worth living and lose interest in healthy lifestyles and healthy eating. In addition, nutritionists have warned about the possibility that isolation will accelerate elderly people's aging and exacerbate FDs further.

1.3 Kaimono-Nanmin (Shopping Refugees) and Food Desert Issues

As mentioned above, there are many so-called 'shuttered streets' (central shopping streets with many closed-down shops or offices) in smaller cities. 'Kaimono-nanmin' (shopping refugees) is a popular expression in Japan. This phrase is usually used in the mass media, such as TV news and newspapers. It means carless elderly people whose homes are close to shuttered streets. They find it difficult to go shopping to distant grocery stores on foot. On the other hand, the government usually uses the term 'Kaimono-jakusya' (disadvantaged shoppers). The Ministry of Economy, Trade and Industry (METI) defines 'Kaimono-jakusya' as elderly people over the age of 60 years who find it difficult to do their daily shopping (Ministry of Economy, Trade and Industry 2010). The definition of 'Kaimono-nanmin' is not clear, but usually both terms have the same meaning. The METI published its report in 2010. In this report, it estimated that the population of Kaimono-jakusya in Japan is approximately six million. The Policy Research Institute of the Ministry of Agriculture, Forestry and

Table 1.1   Estimated population of disadvantaged shoppers in 2015

	Areas	Population over 65 years old (1,000 people)	%
Carless people who live more than 500m from the nearest grocery store	The whole country	8,246	24.6
	Three major metropolitan areas	3,776	23.3
	Tokyo	1,982	23.2
	Nagoya	609	21.5
	Osaka	1,185	24.4
	Provincial areas	4,470	25.9

Source Ministry of Agriculture, Forestry and Fisheries, https://www.maff.go.jp/primaff/seika/fsc/faccess/a_map.html (accessed August 2020)

Fisheries (PRIMAFF) conducted more detailed research in 2011 (Yakushiji 2015) and revised it in 2018. The PRIMAFF calculated the number of carless elderly people over 65 years of age who live more than 500 m from the nearest grocery store. Furthermore, it pointed out that the population of Kaimono-jakusya in Japan is about 8.2 million (Table 1.1).

What is the difference between the Kaimono-nanmin/Kaimono-jakusya issue and the FD issue? The terms 'Kaimono-nanmin' and 'Kaimono-jakusya' describe elderly people's physical problems in their shopping environment (poor food access). In response, the METI has adopted many shopping support policies, such as a subsidy system for so-called shuttered streets, operating vehicle-based mobile shopping services, operating shopping bus services, and disseminating Internet shopping using mobile terminals (tablets). These policies have mainly been implemented in areas of poor food access. In addition, there are many open-air markets and shopping services with residents playing major roles. These new support policies and activities are often reported by the media (for details, please see Chapter 7).

On the other hand, the essence of the FD issue is 'discard the weak.' This is social exclusion. 'FD' is an academic term. Many researchers have analyzed this issue from the perspectives of various academic fields. FD studies are popular in the US, as well as in the UK and other European countries (e.g., Guy 1996; Wrigley et al. 2002; USDA 2012). Many socially vulnerable people are excluded from public services such as educational opportunities, employment opportunities, public health, and safe living environments. FD studies analyze these social exclusion issues through the residents' shopping environment and the opportunity to maintain healthy eating habits. Mr. B, mentioned at the beginning of this chapter, is not a so-called 'Kaimono-nanmin' or 'Kaimono-jakusya' because there are many grocery stores in his neighborhood. However, his local community has lost its closeness. Thus, it is very difficult for him to receive any support from neighbors and maintain his lifestyle, including healthy eating. His neighborhood is not a poor food access area but may be a kind of FD.

In the US and Europe, many patients suffer not only from inconvenient shopping environments but also from a lack of medical facilities, employment, social welfare, and other amenities. There are many factors that cause FD issues in these countries. In Japan, the aging society problem has a severe impact on FD issues. Not only a decrease in the number of nearby stores but also the increase in the number of socially vulnerable people (from the declining birth rate and aging population, limits on welfare, etc.) and decrease in local social capital (weakened ties with families and neighbors) are also major causes of FD issues in Japan. FDs may exist in many places. Even if nearby stores are newly opened, unless the problem of isolation of elderly people remains unresolved, their eating habits will not improve. Poor food access is one factor. We must also attend to the other factors we mentioned above. 'Kaimono-nanmin' and 'Kaimono-jakusya' approaches lack this focus.

1.4   Overseas Research on Food Desert Issues

The term 'food desert' was coined by the British government (Beaumont et al. 1995; Department of Health 1996). It defined FDs as 'those areas of inner cities where cheap nutritious food is virtually unobtainable. Carless residents, unable to reach out-of-town supermarkets, depend on the corner shop where prices are high, products are processed and fresh fruit and vegetables are poor or non-existent' (Whitehead 1998, p. 189).

This social problem has been researched in many academic fields, including geography, nutrition science, and medical science (e.g., Wrigley et al. 2003). For example, economic disparities are a serious social issue in the UK. There is a wide health divide between white-collar workers (relatively high-income people who are usually office workers) and blue-collar workers (relatively low-income people usually engaged in manual labor) (Department of Health 1998; Saul and Payne 1999). Low-income people generally live in the inner-city areas of large cities. Therefore, there is a wide health divide between upper-class residential areas and inner-city areas (Column 1). In the UK, large stores opened one after another on the outskirts of cities from the 1970s to the mid-1990s (Guy 1996). As a result, many individual stores in inner-city areas closed. These commercial changes seriously damaged the living environments of inner-city residents. They could not afford to go to suburban supermarkets, so for daily food they had to depend on corner shops located in inner-city areas that offer little choice (Wrigley et al. 2002). Food in these stores are relatively expensive and they generally do not offer fresh food, such as meat, fish, or vegetables.

There are insufficient social services, such as stores (shopping environments), medical facilities, schools, employment opportunities, or social welfare services, in FDs. The lack of these services, especially the poor shopping environment, often causes poor eating habits (Speak and Graham 1999). Poor eating habits directly damage health. FD studies have started to clarify the reasons for differences in residents' health between regions from the viewpoint of poor food access (hollowing out of central shopping streets).

Although the FD concept is widespread, there is little academic evidence for the actual existence of FDs (Cummins and Macintyre 2002; Smith et al. 2010; Cummins et al. 2010). As mentioned above, diet-related chronic diseases such as obesity have developed in many deprived neighborhoods. Moreover, these areas have universally poorer access to high-quality food environments. A number of studies have analyzed the relationship between poor eating and poor food access and have attempted to prove the existence of FDs. Some before-and-after studies have shown a degree of correlation between access to food and eating behavior. For example, in the UK, a case study conducted in Seacroft, an area of Leeds, showed particular groups of consumers whose diets improved as a result of changing shopping destinations after the opening of new supermarkets in districts with poor food access (Wrigley et al. 2003). However, other studies have been unable to demonstrate any correlation between access to food and eating behavior, and express skepticism regarding the existence of FDs (White et al. 2004; Cummins and Macintyre 2002; Cummins et al. 2010; Smith et al. 2010). However, although a link could not be conclusively proved, some studies have noted that a range of healthy foods is less consistently accessible in some areas, such as remote islands and deprived urban areas (Anderson et al. 2007; Dawson et al. 2007; Smith et al. 2010).

FDs are characterized by deprivation and they compound social exclusion (Wrigley et al. 2002). Although many FD studies primarily address the correlation between limited food access and lower intake of nutritious foods, there may be other explanations for the lower intake. Previous studies have suggested that socioeconomic factors, such as poverty and inadequate knowledge about nutritional benefits, may strongly influence shopping and eating behaviors (Wrigley et al. 2002; Whelan et al. 2002). Thus, not only limited food access, but also soci-economic factors may influence the formation of FDs.

Many studies have addressed FD issues in the US, including a research series by the US Department of Agriculture (USDA) to clarify FD characteristics. For example, the USDA measured access to affordable and nutritious food across North America and analyzed shopping behaviors among low-income residents who live in restricted food access areas (USDA 2009). The USDA defined FDs as census tracts that meet both low-income and low-access criteria (USDA 2012). It then identified 6,529 FD tracts in the US based on the 2000 census and 2006 data on supermarket and large-scale grocery locations. These tracts tended to have residents with lower levels of education, lower income, higher unemployment, and a higher concentration of minority populations. Many other studies, such as those by Weatherspoon et al. (2013, 2015) and Thibodeaux (2015), have also shown that socioeconomic barriers, such as lower income and concentrations of minorities, have a strong influence on shopping behaviors among FD residents (Weatherspoon et al. 2013, 2015; Thibodeaux 2015).

1.5   The Dimensions of Urban Food Desert Studies

The characteristics of FDs (for example, size, location, attributes of victims, and damage caused) are different in each area and country. FD issues are closely related to social exclusion and their backgrounds are complex and different in each country. In Europe and North America, the main victims are low-income people without private cars, represented by foreign workers. East Asian countries, especially Japan, have serious problems with aging populations, which strongly suggests that other barriers to healthy eating by the elderly in Japan give rise to FD issues. It is safe to say that poor food access is one of the major reasons in Japan. However, it is also true that poor food access is not the only reason for Japanese FDs. As mentioned above, we are confident that FD issues are most serious and are expanding in large cities. Many statistical data about elderly people's living environments also support this hypothesis. However, in general, many people believe that 'FDs = poor food access areas = the areas where many disadvantaged shoppers live.' Therefore, urban areas are not the focus of FD studies. It is very difficult to conduct empirical research in urban areas (for example, it is very difficult to conduct questionnaire surveys in big cities because few people respond). This is also a reason why current FD studies disregard urban areas. However, the population is greatest in the central areas of big cities and many voiceless people who suffer from serious FD issues live in these areas.

In this book, we introduce Japanese FD issues. Our case studies are of urban areas. The structure of this book is as follows. In Chapter 2, we present various statistics about elderly people and introduce the Japanese aging problem. In Chapter 3, we explain the two key terms 'food access' and 'ties with families and neighbors' (so-called 'social capital'); these are very important factors in Japanese FD issues. Chapters 4–6 are case studies. In Chapter 4, we present a case study of central Tokyo. Chapter 5 concerns a study of the central areas of a prefectural capital city. Chapter 6 is a case study of a smaller city. In these three chapters, we show the conditions of urban FD issues in Japan. Then, in Chapter 7, we discuss how to solve this problem. In addition, we introduce some noteworthy examples of countermeasures.

Notes

1.   Social capital refers to social networks (ties with people and groups) and normative consciousness based on trust and reciprocity. For more detail, please see Chapter 2, Sect. 2.2.
2.   However, people's eating habits are also influenced by residential areas or national culture (for example, cuisine and manner of eating). Therefore, individual factors are not fully independent of society and are influenced by the living environment to a certain degree.
3.   For example, Aoyama City opened a new commercial complex in the city center in 2001. This building was a symbol of the urban renewal project. However, owing to the lack of customers, this commercial complex soon suffered financial problems and declared bankruptcy in 2017.

References

Anderson AS, Dewar J, Marshall D, Cummins S, Taylor M, Dawson J, Sparks L (2007) The development of a healthy eating indicator shopping basket tool (HEISB) for use in food access studies: identification of key food items. Public Health Nutr 10(12):1440–1447

Arai Y, Hashimoto K (2004) Japanese distribution system and urban space. Kokon Shoin, Tokyo (Japanese)

Beaumont J, Lang T, Leather S, Mucklow C (1995) Report from policy sub-group to the nutrition task force: low income project team. Institute of Grocery Distribution, Watford

Cabinet Office of Japan (2007) National life white paper, 2007 (Japanese). http://www5.cao.go.jp/seikatsu/whitepaper/h19/01_honpen/html/07sh020104.html. Accessed 14 Aug 2020

Cabinet Office of Japan (2015a) White paper on aging society in 2015 (Japanese). http://www8.cao.go.jp/kourei/whitepaper/w-2015/zenbun/pdf/1s1s_2.pdf. Accessed 14 Aug 2020

Cabinet Office of Japan (2015b) Public opinion research on social consciousness (Japanese). http://survey.gov-online.go.jp/h25/h25-shakai/. Accessed 14 Aug 2020

Cummins S, Macintyre S (2002) Food deserts: evidence and assumption in health policy making. BMJ 325(7361):436–438

Cummins S, Smith DM, Aitken Z, Dawson J, Marshall D, Spark L, Anderson AS (2010) Neighbourhood deprivation and the price and availability of fruit and vegetables in Scotland. J Hum Nutr Diet 23:494–501

Dawson J, Marshall D, Taylor M, Cummins S, Sparks L, Anderson A (2007) Accessing healthy food: a sentinel mapping study of healthy food retailing in Scotland. Executive Summary. Food Standards Agency (Scotland), Aberdeen. http://www.food.gov.uk/sites/default/files/multimedia/pdfs/publication/accessinghealthyfood0108.pdf#search='accessing+healthy+food+a+sentinel+mapping+study+of+healthy+food+retailing+in+scotland'. Accessed 14 Aug 2020

Department of Health (1996) Low income, food, nutrition and health: strategies for improvement. In: A report from the low-income project to the nutrition task force. Department of Health, London

Department of Health (1998) Nutritional aspects of the development of cancer. The Stationery Office, London

European Commission, Environment (1990) Green paper on the urban environment: environment and quality of life: environment and quality of life, 27 June 1990. EU Commission—COM Document. http://aei.pitt.edu/1205/. Accessed 14 Aug 2020

Guy CM (1996) Corporate strategies in food retailing and their local impacts: a case study of Cardiff. Environ Plan A 28(9):1575–1602

Hirayama Y (2006) The edge of Tokyo. NTT Publishing Co., Ltd, Tokyo (Japanese)

Iwama N (ed) (2011) Food desert issues: food deserts and isolated society. Association of Agriculture and Forestry Statistics, Tokyo (Japanese)

Iwama N (ed) (2013) Newly revised edition: food desert issues: food deserts and isolated society. Association of Agriculture and Forestry Statistics, Tokyo (Japanese)

Iwama N (ed) (2017) Urban food deserts issues: urban food deserts in low-social capital areas. Association of Agriculture and Forestry Statistics, Tokyo (Japanese)

Kaido K (2001) Compact city. Gakugei Shuppansha, Tokyo (Japanese)

Kikushima R, Takahashi K (2018) Effects of shopping service on dietary diversity: analysis of MAFF's questionnaire survey on awareness of food access. J Food Syst Res 29:29–42 (Japanese with English abstract)

Kondo K (2007) Health disparity society: social epidemiological large research study towards care prevention. Igaku Shoin, Tokyo (Japanese)

Kumagai S (2011) Stop poor eating habits: nutrition for healthy life. Kodainsha, Tokyo (Japanese)

Ministry of Economy, Trade and Industry (2010) Research report on distribution system to support local life infrastructure (Japanese). http://www.meti.go.jp/report/downloadfiles/g100514a03j.pdf. Accessed 14 Aug 2020

Ministry of Internal Affairs and Communications (2019) Annual Report on the Ageing Society. https://www8.cao.go.jp/kourei/english/annualreport/2019/pdf/2019.pdf. Accessed 9 Mar 2021

Ohashi M, Takahashi K, Kikushima R, Yamaguchi M, Yakushiji T (2017) The effect of food access on elderly women's food consumption and health: results of mail surveys from the City Center of Shirakawa, Fukushima, Japan. J Food Syst Res 24(2):61–71 (Japanese with English abstract)

Saul C, Payne N (1999) How does the prevalence of specific morbidities compare with measures of socioeconomic status and at small area level? J Public Health Med 21:340–347

Smith DM, Cummins S, Taylor M, Dawson J, Marshall D, Sparks L, Anderson AS (2010) Neighbourhood food environment and area deprivation: spatial accessibility to grocery stores selling fresh fruit and vegetables in urban and rural settings. Int J Epidemiol 39(1):277–284

Speak S, Graham S (1999) Service not included: private services restructuring, neighbourhoods, and social marginalization. Environ Plan A 31(11):1985–2001

Thibodeaux J (2015) City racial composition as a predictor of African American food deserts. Urban Stud 53(11):2238–2252

US Department of Agriculture (2009) Access to affordable and nutritious food: measuring and understanding food deserts and their consequences. http://www.ers.usda.gov/publications/ap-administrative-publication/ap-036.aspx. Accessed 14 Aug 2020

US Department of Agriculture (2012) Characteristics and influential factors of food deserts. http://www.ers.usda.gov/publications/err-economic-research-report/err140.aspx. Accessed 14 Aug 2020

Weatherspoon D, Oehmke J, Dembele A, Coleman M, Satimanon T, Weatherspoon L (2013) Price and expenditure elasticities for fresh fruits in an urban food desert. Urban Stud 50(1):88–106

Weatherspoon D, Oehmke J, Dembele A, Weatherspoon L (2015) Fresh vegetable demand behaviour in an urban food desert. Urban Stud 52(5):960–979

Whelan A, Wrigley N, Warm D, Cannings E (2002) Life in a 'food desert'. Urban Stud 39(11):2083–2100

White M, Bunting J, Raybauld S, Adamson A, Williams I, Mathers J (2004) Do food deserts exist? A multi-level geographical analysis of the relationship between retail food access, socio-economic position and dietary intake. Final report to Food Standards Agency. www.ncl.ac.uk/ihs/assets/pdfs/fsareport.pdf#search='Do+food+deserts+exist%3F+A+multilevel+geographical+analysis'. Accessed 14 Aug 2020

Whitehead M (1998) Food deserts: what's in a name? Health Educ J 57:189–190

Wrigley N, Warm D, Margetts B (2003) Deprivation, diet, and food-retail access: findings from the Leeds 'food deserts' study. Environ Plan A 35:151–188

Wrigley N, Warm D, Margetts B, Whelan A (2002) Assessing the impact of improved retailed access of diet in a 'food desert': a preliminary report. Urban Stud 39:2061–2082

Yagi K, Takahashi K, Kikushima R, Yamaguchi M, Oura Y, Tamaki, Yamamoto J (2019) Food consumption patterns and nutrient intake among adult men in tokyo metropolitan area. J Food Syst Res 26(1): 2–11 (Japanese with English abstract)

Yakushiji T (2015) Food access issues in an elderly society. Harvest Publishing Co. Ltd, Tokyo (Japanese)

Chapter 2
The Background of Japanese Food Desert Issues

Abstract In this chapter, we explain the socioeconomic background of Japanese FDs in terms of the increase in the number of socially vulnerable people and their distribution in Tokyo. Japan has the most rapidly aging society in the world, and its declining birth rate is also remarkable. The elderly person are main sufferers of Japanese Food deserts (FDs). Changes in the environment associated with retailing and distribution have a significant influence on FDs. The diversification of the population structure in central Tokyo also deteriorates elderly person's living environments. The elderly residents of central Tokyo share their living environment with this variety of people. In these areas, it is difficult to construct a mutual assistance system. These are major factors in the expansion of the FD problem in this gigantic city.

Keywords The socioeconomic background of Japanese food desert issues · Socially vulnerable people · Aging society · The diversification of the population structure

2.1 Background of the Japanese Food Desert Issue

In Japan, the Food Desert (FD) issue arose at the beginning of the 2000s. Why has the FD issue recently become more serious? To answer this question, we must explain specific Japanese socioeconomic conditions. In this chapter, we explain the background of Japanese FDs in terms of (1) the increase in the number of socially vulnerable people (Sect. 2.1) and (2) their distribution in Tokyo (Sect. 2.2). Figure 2.1 shows the important factors in the occurrence of FD issues in each area (Iwama 2017).

2.1.1 The Increasing Elderly Population

Japan has the most rapidly aging society in the world, and its declining birth rate is also remarkable. The total population is 126,434,565 people, of whom approximately 28.1% are over 65 years of age (December 2018). The overall Japanese fertility rate is 1.42 children per woman. This rate is the lowest in the world after Korea (0.98)

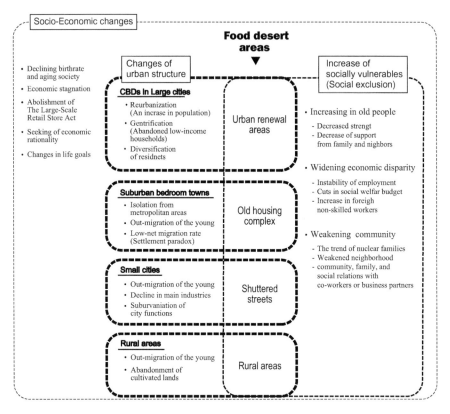

Fig. 2.1 Factors of Japanese food desert issues. *Source* Iwama ed. (2011) (partially revised)

and Taiwan (1.13). East Asia is an aging region and this tendency is remarkable in Japan. In relation to shopping activities, it is very difficult for an elderly person to travel long distances on foot or by bicycle. In addition, many people receive too little support from family members because of the nuclearization of the family. We discuss the decreasing birthrate and aging population in the next section.

2.1.2 Environmental Changes Associated with Retailing and Distribution

Changes in the environment associated with retailing and distribution also have a significant influence on FDs. Drastic spatial structural transformation in metropolitan areas and distribution systems has changed urban retailing systems (Arai and Hashimoto 2004). In particular, the deregulation of large stores has had a significant influence on urban retailing systems. The *Large Retail Store Law*, which took effect in 1974, was intended to secure appropriate opportunities for small–medium retailers' business activities and strictly regulate large stores' activities. Mom-and-Pop stores were protected by this law for a long time. However, because of pressure from foreign countries seeking to enter the Japanese market and strong criticism of overprotectiveness of small retailers, the Japanese government softened this law gradually in the 1990s and completely abolished it in 2000. Now, the so-called three town development laws—the *Large Retail Store Location Law,* the *Urban Planning Act* (revised 2006), and the *Law on Improvement and Revitalization of City Centers*—have been in force since 2000. The *Large Retail Store Location Law* is to maintain the living environment of the residents around large stores, and it is less strict in relation to large retailers compared with the *Large Retail Store Law.* In addition, such regulations outside cities are less strict. Therefore, the number of large stores has rapidly increased in suburban areas since deregulation. The deregulation also hollowed out central shopping streets (Yahagi 2005; Yamakawa 2004). The total number of retail stores in Japan was 1,721,465 in 1982 (at the peak), but the total number of retail stores in 2016 was 990,249 (1982 Commercial Statistics and 2016 Economic Census). On the other hand, the total floor space of retail stores has increased ($95,430,071 \, m^2$ in 1982 to $135,343,693 \, m^2$ in 2016). These data suggest that although many small retailers have been bankrupted, many large retailers, including supermarkets, have opened. In addition, the Japanese retail market has shrunk since 1997 and this economic environment led many small retailers into bankruptcy too.

Current social systems seeking economic rationality also have a significant influence on Japanese FDs. Many retail chains and public bus companies withdraw their businesses from low profitability areas, including rural villages and small towns, and these changes expand areas with poor social services. For example, the reduction of government subsidies in 2001 and deregulation of bus businesses in 2002 have made it easy for many companies to enter and withdraw from the public bus business. As a result, many companies closed their operations in rural areas. Some of these municipalities cannot provide any alternatives yet. Discussions must be held on public transport services in unprofitable rural areas.

2.1.3 The Expansion of Poverty

The increase in the number of low-income families is also a major cause of FD issues. Japan was called an "all-middle-class society" from the 1970s to the 1990s. However, economic inequality is now increasing. The proportion of families in relative poverty (with an equivalent disposable income of less than half of the overall median) in 1985 was 12% but increased to 15.6% in 2015 (Ministry of Health, Labour and Welfare 2017). The Japanese poverty ratio is the second lowest among the G7 nations. The average disposable income of families in relative poverty in Japan is 1.22 million yen in 2015. The poverty ratio is higher for single parent families and the elderly.

The elderly exhibit a trend toward polarization. On one hand, many elderly people are rich in assets. However, on the other, many poor elderly people must depend only on their basic pension from the government to cover all their expenses.

Usually, those over 65 years of age receive both a basic pension and a second-tier pension (e.g., a welfare pension or a mutual pension). However, people without full-time jobs, with an independent business, or whose employers have not paid a premium for their employees cannot receive a second-tier pension after retirement. The basic pension is about 60,000 yen per month for a single-person household, and 130,000 yen for a couple. In fact, the basic pension is insufficient to live on, but 11.9 million people depend on this alone (Social Insurance Agency 2007). Moreover, a person in arrears of the national pension cannot obtain even a basic pension. About 3.2 million people receive no pension from the government (Ministry of Health, Labour and Welfare 2008). A reduction in the nursing care budget has also had a serious effect on low-income people's daily lives.

2.1.4 The Weakening of Families and Local Communities

Changes in life goals is also a significant factor in the increased numbers of socially vulnerable people. In the 60 years since the end of World War 2, the general goals in Japanese people's lives have changed such as: "escape from poverty" (1945–early 1970s), "the attainment of an average living standard" (late 1970s–1980s), and "the era of diversification" (since the 1990s) (Hirayama 2006). In former times, people generally desired to achieve standard life goals, including employment, marriage, and children. However, these are no longer general goals. Because of the diversity of values, the number of people who do not desire employment, marriage, or children is increasing. The increase in the unemployment rate, the expansion of income inequality, and uncertainty about the future have accelerated the rate of changes in standard life goals. As a result, the proportion of single households has recently increased rapidly (for more detail, please see Sect. 2.2). These changes often weaken ties with families and tend to encourage the corruption existing in support systems by family members.

The weakening of local communities is also remarkable. In 1975, 85.6% of Japanese people reported that "I usually communicate with neighbors" and only 1.5% that "I do not communicate with neighbors." However, in 2017, the proportion reporting that "I usually communicate with neighbors (I have a relationship with neighbors)" was 67.7% and that of "I do not communicate with neighbors" was 32.14% (Cabinet Office 1975, 2007). The weakening of local communities is more remarkable in urban areas (Shiga University and Cabinet Office 2016). The main reasons for weakened ties within local communities are such as: "many people do not stay in my house in daytime and they rarely meet neighbors," "the Parent–Teacher Association is one of the most important local community activities. But because of the decrease in the birth rate, this association is inactive compared with before," and because residents move frequently, local people's attachments to their place of residence are decreasing (the diversity of residents, residents' mobility) (Ministry of Land, Infrastructure and Transport 2007).

2.1.5 The Diversity of Residents

The diversity of urban residents is also remarkable (for more detail, please see Sect. 2.2). The floating population is large in big cities. Therefore, many people from many places, including those from overseas, live in the same districts. Their social attributes are also diverse. They include elderly people, technical specialists, single professionals (especially career women), and university students. A wide variety of people live in big cities as neighbors. The globalization of residents is also remarkable, and the number of expatriates is also increasing. The number of medium- and long-term expatriates in June 2018 was 2,637,251 (2.09% of the total population), and more than half of these are from Asia. This proportion in 1990 was 1,075,313 (0.87% of the total population). Therefore, it is safe to say that the number of expatriates is also increasing rapidly. Many of these people live in big cities. As we discuss in Sect. 2.2, the diversity of residents often prevents local communities from creating intimate relationships.

2.2 Population Aging and the Diversification of the Population Structure in Central Tokyo

2.2.1 Changes in the Population Structure with a Declining Birthrate and an Aging Population

In this chapter, population aging and the diversification of the population structure in the central part of Tokyo, which underlie the FD problem, are analyzed using statistical data. Because of a prolonged economic recession, a declining birthrate, and an aging population, the lives of elderly people became harder because of problems such as pension issues and reductions in medical insurance. These days, human relationships are also becoming poorer not only for elderly people but also for the younger generation. In this chapter, we describe the current state of Japanese society and analyze the root causes of the FD problem. In addition, we predict the future population and examine the question of which regions will suffer from population aging in the future.

2.2.1.1 Changes in Population by Age Group

First, we attempt to describe Japanese society with its declining birthrate and aging population by dividing the population according to age group. Figure 2.2 shows population age groups in a vertical bar graph. The values in the graph are values from 1935 to 2010, with estimated values from 2015 to 2050. The young population (0–14 years), the working age population (15–64 years), the elderly (65–74 years),

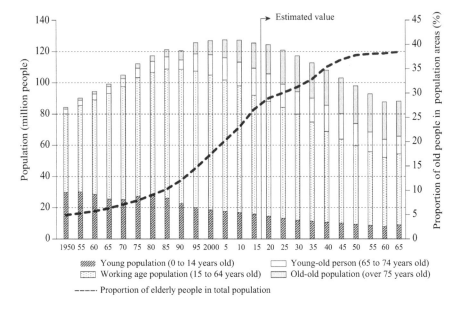

Fig. 2.2 Population by age groups. *Source* National Institute of Population and Social Security Research (2021)

and the very elderly (over 75 years old) were used as age groups. The proportion of elderly people in the population is shown as a line graph.

The young population increased after 1935, and it was about 30 million in 1955. After that, it decreased consistently until 2005, and it is expected to continue decreasing until 2050. As a result, the total population will peak at about 128 million in 2005, and then it is expected to decrease consistently.

On the other hand, the proportion of elderly people exceeded 7% in 1970; it was said that aging had begun in the Japanese society. As this proportion exceeded 14% in 1995, it was said that the aging society had come. As it passed 21% in 2010, the media reported that Japan had become a super-aging society.

However, it is necessary to pay attention to the significance of the values of 7, 14, and 21%. The UN's definition of an aging society is one in which the elderly population exceeds 7% of the total. However, there was no scientific basis for this definition. "This definition was used for the time being with reference to the demographic structure of advanced countries at that time" (Tsuji 2003). A value of 7% should not be an absolute standard. Similarly, a value of 14% has no meaning beyond being twice that of 7%.

What should be noted more is that the number of very elderly people has increased owing to increased life expectancy. In 2010, the number of elderly people was 1.5 million and that of very elderly people was 1.4 million; the numbers were almost the same. However, in 2020, the number of elderly people is estimated to be 1.7 million and that of very elderly people, 1.9 million; the number of very elderly people is expected to continue to exceed the number of elderly people. Very elderly people are at greater risk of health and living problems than other elderly people. Therefore, the number of elderly people facing many living problems is expected to increase. One such problem is FD.

2.2.1.2 Changes in Age Structure

Figure 2.2 shows the population divided by age group. It shows the young population ratio which is the ratio of young people under 14 years old to the total population, and the elderly in the population, which is the ratio of people over 65 years old to the total population. It also shows the young age dependency ratio, which is the ratio of young people in the population to the working age population (15–64 years old) of 100 people and the old age dependency ratio, which is the ratio of elderly people to the working age population of 100 people. The index of aging is the ratio of elderly to 100 young people. Figure 2.3 shows these five line graphs. The values in the line graphs are those recorded between 1935 and 2010, with projected values for 2015–2050.

The young population ratio peaked at about 40% in 1935, and then decreased consistently until 2010. This value is expected to decline further after 2015. On the other hand, the old age dependency ratio was 4.7% in 1935 and 7.1% in 1970. This

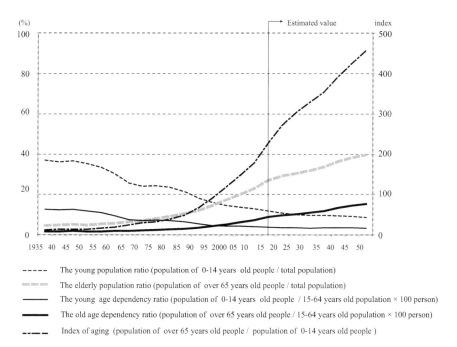

----- The young population ratio (population of 0-14 years old people / total population)

▬ ▬ ▬ The elderly population ratio (population of over 65 years old people / total population)

——— The young age dependency ratio (population of 0-14 years old people / 15-64 years old population × 100 person)

━━━ The old age dependency ratio (population of over 65 years old people / 15-64 years old population × 100 person)

━ ━ ━ Index of aging (population of over 65 years old people / population of 0-14 years old people)

Fig. 2.3 Indexes about age structure. *Source* National Institute of Population and Social Security Research (2021)

value rose only 2.4 points in 35 years. However, it rose 13 points in the following 35 years; it was 20.1% in 2005. This value is expected to increase further after 2010 and is expected to reach 36.1% in 2040.

The young population is comprised of those under 14 years old, who cannot work. The elderly are those over 65 years old, who are expected to retire from the labor market. The age group that can participate in the labor market is the working age population over 15 and under 65 years old. The young age dependency ratio, which is the ratio of the young people to 100 working age people, was 63.1% in 1935. This means that 10 people of working age had to support six young people at that time. However, this value is expected to reach 20.7 in 2010 and decline to 18.8 in 2050. Therefore, it is expected that 10 people of working age will support two young people in 2050. In contrast, the old age dependency ratio is 36.1% in 2010 and is expected to reach 75.3% in 2050. Ten working age people must currently support four elderly people, and this figure will reach eight elderly people in 2050.

The index of aging, which is the ratio of elderly people to 100 young people, was 119.1 in 2000. It is expected to exceed 200 in 2015, 300 in 2030, and 400 in 2050. In 2015, the number of elderly people is expected to be double that of children, triple in 2030, and four times the number in 2050. This is the structure of Japanese society in the future.

2.2.2   Aging and the Dilution of Family Relationships in the Generation of Demographic Transition

2.2.2.1   The Generation of Demographic Transition

To predict changes in the living environment of the elderly, it is necessary to see the changes in family structure. Figure 2.4 shows the change in the population pyramid from 1930 to 2050.

The population pyramid is a diagram of the number of males in each age group on the left and the number of females on the right. The population pyramids from 1930 and 1950 show the patterns of natality and mortality.

In demography, the generation born between 1925 and 1950 is said to be the generation of demographic transition. The generation born between 1947 and 1949 is called the "baby boomer" generation. The population pyramid for 1960–1990 shows many children of the baby boomer generation; however, the size of the other generations is declining. The generation born between 1925 and 1950 grew up in large families, but they made nuclear families. This social change is the reason why this generation is called the generation of demographic transition.

The decline in birthrate and population aging are expected to continue after 2010. Figure 2.5 shows the number of households by family type. Figure 2.6 shows that the proportion of single elderly person households will increase. Therefore, there is

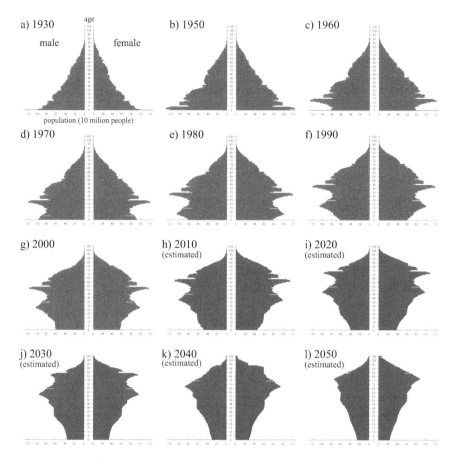

Fig. 2.4 Change in the population pyramid from 1930 to 2050. *Source* National Institute of Population and Social Security Research (2021)

a high probability that extended families will rapidly disappear. This means that it will be difficult for extended families to function as safety nets for elderly people.

2.2.2.2 Moving to a Big City

Where does the generation of demographic transition live? This question will be answered with an analysis of a cohort share. Oe (2003) showed the nationwide share of each cohort and each age group in the Tokyo metropolitan area, comprised of Tokyo, Kanagawa, Saitama, and Chiba. Of the people born between 1931 and 1935, 15% lived in the Tokyo metropolitan area when they were under five years of age. When this cohort was 20–24 years old, about 20% lived there. When the cohort was

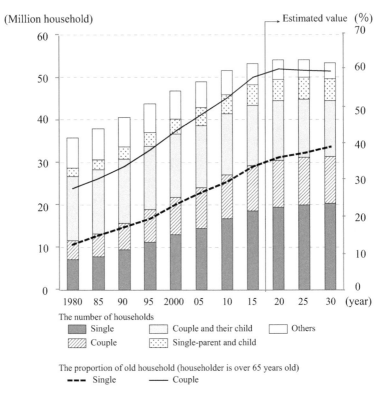

Fig. 2.5 Number of households by family type from 1980 to 2030. *Source* National Institute of Population and Social Security Research (2021) (partly revised)

35–39 years old, about 23% lived there. After that, the proportion living in Tokyo remained the same.

Figure 2.6 shows that about 25% of the generation of demographic transition were concentrated in the Tokyo metropolitan area between the ages of 15 and 24 and remained thereafter. About 23% of the next generation were concentrated in the Tokyo metropolitan area after they were born, so the second generation was born in Tokyo. More people of this generation were concentrated in the Tokyo metropolitan area when they were 15–24 years old; 30% of them lived there.

Therefore, the generation of demographic transition was born in big families, moved to big cities, and raised their children in nuclear families.

2.2.2.3 Movement Within the Tokyo Metropolitan Area

The movements of baby boomers, who were the last generation of the generation of demographic transition, within the metropolitan area were analyzed using a social atlas. A population census is conducted every five years. The proportions of each

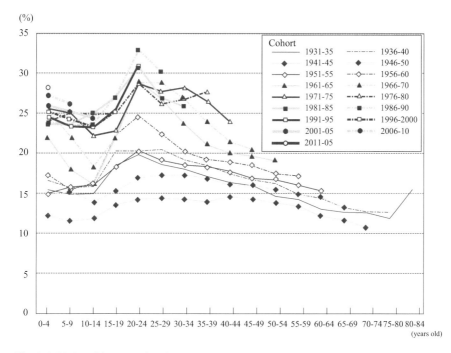

Fig. 2.6 Nationwide share of each cohot and age group on Tokyo metropolitan area. *Source* Oe (2003) (partly revised)

age group, including baby boomers, in the total population are shown in Fig. 2.7 (Kurasawa and Asakawa 2004).

This generation was 20–24 years old in 1970. Figure 2.7a shows baby boomers concentrated in the Tokyo metropolitan area, which means that the younger baby boomers moved towards the center of Tokyo where there were many opportunities for study and work.

The areas where the proportion of this generation was high moved slightly to include some suburbs in 1975. They turned 30–34 years old and reached the life stage to give birth and raise children by 1980. The proportion of baby boomers in 23 wards declined, but that in the suburbs increased. Suburbanization continued until 1990.

Figures 2.4, 2.5, 2.6, and 2.7 show that the generation of demographic transition moved into the central part of Tokyo and then to the suburbs. Therefore, the numbers of single elderly people and couples have increased in the suburbs.

The suburbs have smaller populations than the center, and the central part of the city has the most elderly people. It is necessary to note this point.

a) 1970   20-24 years old
   :from local cities to Tokyo

b) 1975   25-29 years old
   :from Tokyo to suburban areas

c) 1980   30-34 years old

d) 1990   40-44 years old

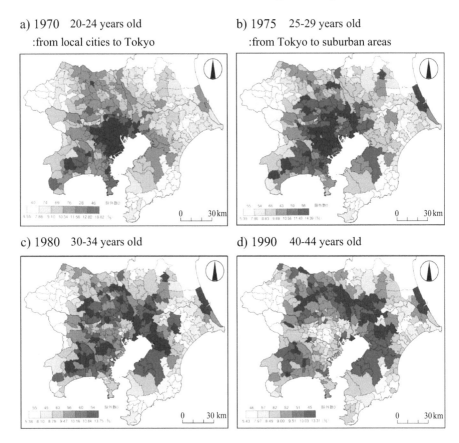

Fig. 2.7 Residential movement of Baby-Boom Generation in Tokyo metropolitan area. *Source* Kurasawa and Asakawa (2004)

2.2.3 Diversity of the Population Structure in the City Center

So far, the overall population structure of Japan in the past, present, and future has been described. Local communities in Japan vary. Some local communities have large populations and others have smaller populations, which face the risk of disappearing altogether. Therefore, in the next part, local communities will be analyzed using the 2010 population census. The unit of analysis was a third mesh (a third-order grid of about 1 km square), and the area for analysis was that within a 60 km radius of the Tokyo station. The six class classifications were calculated from the average and standard deviation.

Figure 2.8 shows that the proportion of elderly people is low in the center of the city and higher at the periphery. However, although few elderly people live in Chiyoda

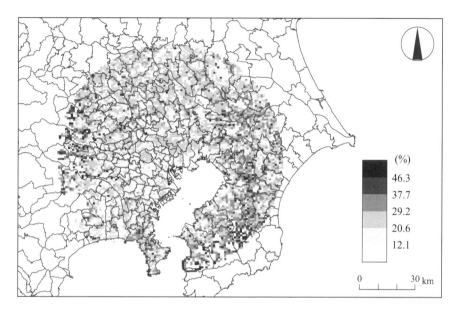

Fig. 2.8 Elderly population ratio in Tokyo metropolitan area in 2010. *Source* Population Census (2010)

ward, more than 1,000 live in each square kilometer. The meshes with more than 1,000 elderly people are spread over 23 wards (Fig. 2.9). Because many people live in the central part of the city, the proportion of elderly people has become relatively low. However, it is necessary to keep in mind that many elderly people live there.

Next, the structure of elderly people's households will be shown. Figure 2.10 shows the proportion of single elderly households, which exceeds 10% in Tokyo's 23 wards. The number of single elderly households in the one-kilometer square mesh exceeds 400. On the other hand, the proportion of elderly couple households in Tokyo's 23 wards is low, but high in the area surrounding the 23 wards (Fig. 2.11). Both ratios were low in the southern part of Ibaraki. This means that many people live in their children's households in these areas.

A high proportion of professional technical workers live in the central part of Tokyo. Male professional technical workers live along the Chuo, Odakyu, and Keisei railway lines in the western part of the 23 wards (Fig. 2.12). In contrast, female professional technical workers live in the eastern part, such as the Chuo or Koto wards (Fig. 2.13). The figure shows that highly educated white-collar females are relatively concentrated in the central part of Tokyo.

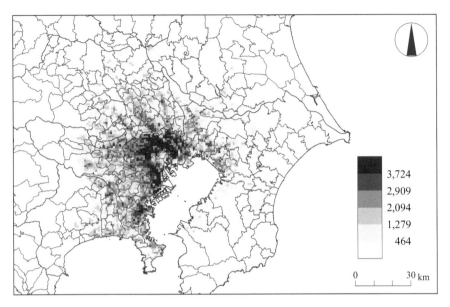

Fig. 2.9 Population of old people over 65 years in Tokyo metropolitan area in 2010. *Source*
Population Census (2010)

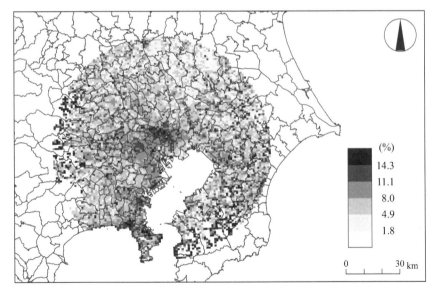

Fig. 2.10 Proportion of single elderly household in Tokyo metropolitan area in 2010. *Source*
Population Census (2010)

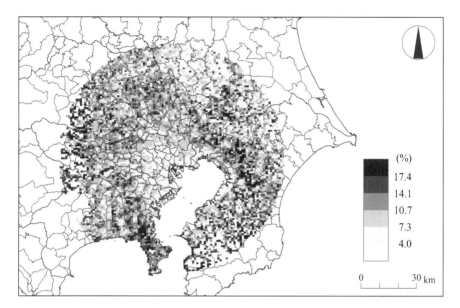

Fig. 2.11 Proportion of elderly couple household in Tokyo metropolitan area in 2010. *Source* Population Census (2010)

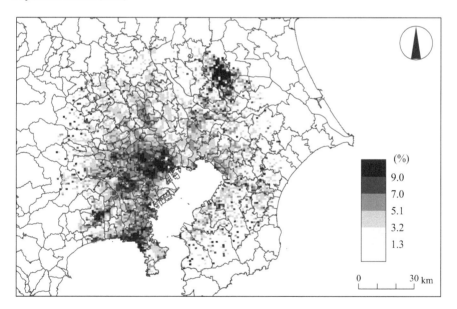

Fig. 2.12 Proportion of professional technical workers in Tokyo metropolitan area in 2010. *Source* Population Census (2010)

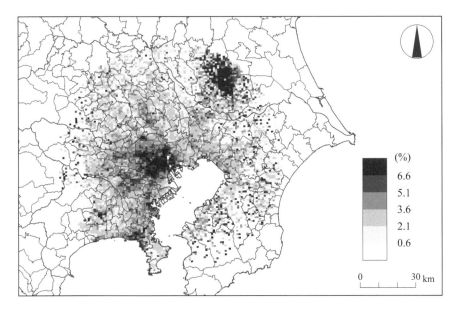

Fig. 2.13 Proportion of female professional technical workers in Tokyo metropolitan area in 2010. *Source* Population Census (2010)

However, it is not only the highly educated and high-income people that live in central Tokyo. Figure 2.14 shows the unemployment rate. The unemployment rate in the western part of Tokyo's 23 wards is relatively low. There is high unemployment in parts of the Nakano and Shinjuku wards. In the north-eastern part of the 23 wards, the unemployment rate is relatively high. Figure 2.15 shows high proportions of public housing in the northern part, eastern part, bay area, and western suburbs of the 23 wards. These social atlases show that not all people living in the center of Tokyo are rich.

As mentioned above, there are many single elderly people in the center of Tokyo. Nevertheless, the proportion of households of single people in their 20s is also high (Fig. 2.16). Younger people are attracted to the center of Tokyo because of its opportunities for study, work, and housing. For similar reasons, there are also many foreigners. Figure 2.17 shows the ratio of foreign people per 1000 population. This figure shows that the proportion of foreign people in the 23 wards is higher than that in Kawasaki and Yokohama cities, where many foreigners are concentrated.

From the above results, the population structure of central Tokyo is described as follows. (1) It is diverse. (2) Many single elderly people live there. (3) There are many households of single people in their 20s, as well as highly educated white-collar females and foreigners.

The elderly residents of central Tokyo share their living environment with this variety of people. In these areas, it is difficult to construct a mutual assistance system. This is a major factor in the expansion of the FD problem in this gigantic city.

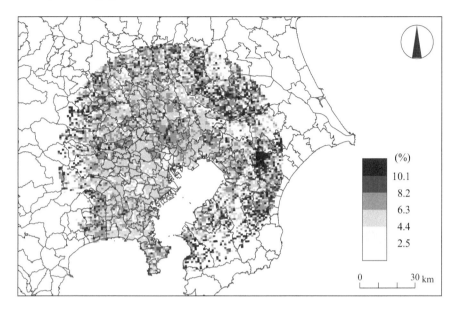

Fig. 2.14 Unemployment rate in Tokyo metropolitan area in 2010. *Source* Population Census (2010)

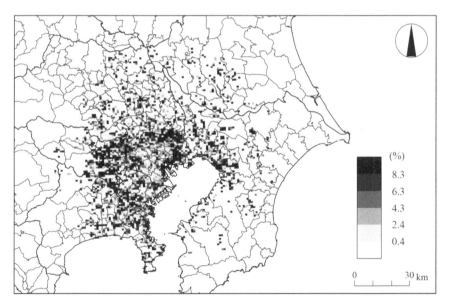

Fig. 2.15 Proportion of public housing residents in Tokyo metropolitan area in 2010. *Source* Population Census (2010)

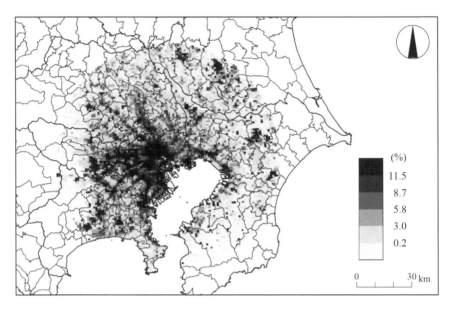

Fig. 2.16 Proportion of household of single people in their 20s in Tokyo metropolitan area in 2010. *Source* Population Census (2010)

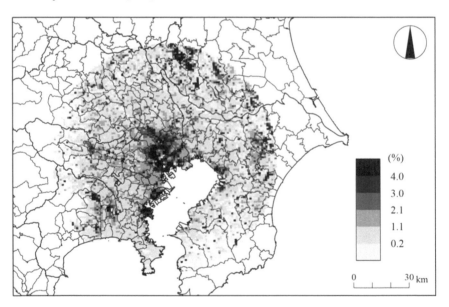

Fig. 2.17 Proportion of foreign people per 1000 population in Tokyo metropolitan area in 2010. *Source* Population Census (2010)

References

Arai Y, Hashimoto K (2004) The distribution and urban space in Japan. Kokon Shoin, Tokyo (Japanese)

Cabinet Office (1975) The national survey on lifestyle preferences. Cabinet Office, Tokyo (Japanese)

Cabinet Office (2007) An opinion poll. Cabinet Office, Tokyo (Japanese)

Hirayama Y (2006) The end of Tokyo. NTT publishing Co. Ltd, Tokyo (Japanese)

Iwama N (ed) (2011) Food desert issues: food deserts and isolated society. Association of Agriculture and Forestry Statistics, Tokyo (Japanese)

Iwama N (ed) (2017) Urban food deserts issues: urban food deserts in low-social capital areas. Association of Agriculture and Forestry Statistics, Tokyo (Japanese)

Kurasawa S, Asakawa T (eds) (2004) The social maps of Tokyo metropolitan area. University of Tokyo Press, Tokyo (Japanese)

Ministry of Health, Labour and Welfare (2008) Comprehensive survey of living conditions in 2007 (Japanese). http://www.wam.go.jp/wamappl/bb14GS50.nsf/0/5D7C0BC46310507949257 4C100019893?OpenDocument. Accessed 14 Aug 2020

Ministry of Health, Labour and Welfare (2017) Comprehensive survey of living conditions in 2017 (Japanese). https://www.mhlw.go.jp/toukei/saikin/hw/k-tyosa/k-tyosa17/index.html. Accessed 14 Aug 2020

Ministry of Land, Infrastructure and Transport (2007) White book on land, infrastructure, transport and tourism in Japan. http://www.mlit.go.jp/hakusyo/mlit/index.html (Japanese). Accessed 14 Aug 2020

National Institute of Population and Social Security Research (2021) http://www.ipss.go.jp/. Accessed 9 Mar 2021

Oe M (2003) Population change and urban housing policy. In: Okabe M (ed) The frontier of policy studies: market/risk/sustainability. Keio University Press, Tokyo, pp 194–220 (Japanese)

Population Census (2010) https://www.stat.go.jp/data/kokusei/2010/. Accessed 9 Mar 2021

Shiga University and Cabinet Office (2016) Local revitalization using rich social capital (Japanese). http://www.esri.go.jp/jp/prj/hou/hou075/hou75.pdf. Accessed 14 Aug 2020

Social Insurance Agency (2007) An outline of the social insurance business in 2006 (Japanese). http://www.mhlw.go.jp/topics/bukyoku/nenkin/nenkin/toukei/dl/h18a.pdf#search='%E5%B9% B3%E6%88%9018%E5%B9%B4%E5%BA%A6%E7%A4%BE%E4%BC%9A%E4%BF% 9D%E9%99%BA%E4%BA%8B%E6%A5%AD%E3%81%AE%E6%A6%82%E6%B3%81'. Accessed 14 Aug 2020

Tsuji A (2003) Aging of population. In: Koyano T, Ando T (eds) Revised edition: new socio-gerontology. World Pannning Co, Ltd, Tokyo (Japanese), pp 27–54

Yahagi H (2005) Large store and urban development. Iwanami Shinsho, Tokyo (Japanese)

Yamakawa M (2004) Large stores and redevelopment of shopping streets. Hukushima University, Hukushima (Japanese)

Chapter 3
Food Access and Social Capital

Abstract As mentioned in Chapter 1, we hypothesized that food access (i.e. the distance between homes and the nearest grocery stores) and local social capital (SC; i.e. ties with family and neighbors) are the most important factors in the occurrence of food desert (FD) issues in Japan. SC plays an especially important role in urban FDs. Food access and local SC (discussed below) are geographical (i.e. living environment) factors, and FD is a geographical issue. To identify FD locations, we must measure factors statistically. In this chapter, we introduce how to measure food access (Sect. 3.1) and local SC (Sect. 3.2).

Keywords Food access · Food desert · Social capital · Measurement method · Geographic information system

3.1 Introduction

A primary purpose of this book is to create a food desert (FD) map, which will help us understand FD issues. In addition, because this map might clarify the locations of elderly adults who suffer from FD problems and need support, this map may facilitate preventative care for socially vulnerable people. To create a highly accurate FD map, we must measure food access and social capital (SC) in each research area. There are ways to measure food access and SC; thus, in this chapter, we introduce these techniques in Sects. 3.1 and 3.2, respectively.

3.2   Measurement of Food Access and Making Food Access Maps

3.2.1   Measuring Food Access and Mapping People with Limited Access to Shopping Facilities

3.2.1.1   Statistical Data on People with Limited Access to Shopping Facilities

The number of people who feel they have trouble shopping can be estimated using a questionnaire survey with sufficient sample size. As mentioned in Chapter 1, a report by the Study Group on the Role of Distribution Systems in Community Infrastructure for the Ministry of Economy, Trade and Industry (METI) published in May 2010 found that approximately six million people have limited access to shopping facilities in Japan. The basis for this figure was a report commissioned by the Cabinet Office and conducted in 2005 titled *Results of Survey on Senior Citizens' Attitude toward Housing and the Living Environment* and based on a web questionnaire. The ministry announced that the number of vulnerable shoppers increased to about seven million in April 2015.

The estimated values based on these questionnaires depend on respondents' subjective evaluations. The objective standard for those with limited access to shopping facilities is not shown. In addition, the questionnaire survey method—based on sampling—does not reveal the places where many feel shopping is inconvenient, although this number can be estimated. To address FD problems with specific measures, spatial information on where and how they arise is indispensable. Unless we know the areas where FD problems occur, we cannot consider specific services such as mobile vending vehicles and food distribution.

The Food Access Map of the Ministry of Agriculture, Forestry and Fisheries Policy Research Institute (PRIMAFF) introduced in Chapter 1 makes it possible to ascertain the ease of access to grocery stores in Japan by browsing the Internet. However, this map is based on an area-wide mesh (a fourth-order grid of about 500 m square), and it is impossible to know the exact location of a store in the grid. Therefore, to clarify food access at the block level, it is necessary to accurately determine store locations.

An area with many people who have limited access to shopping facilities can be mapped in several ways using existing maps and population data. The following sections explain several of these methods.

3.2.1.2   How to Create Poor Food Access Maps

In recent years, digital data in forms such as maps and statistics have become easily available through the Internet. Therefore, even without special technology or software, simple food access can be measured with a map and pen based on those data.

In addition, a Geographic Information System (GIS) can be used to measure food access and map FD risk areas more accurately.

This section introduces how to create poor food access maps. To identify areas with large numbers of people, it is necessary to measure the balance between demand for, and supply of, fresh food. In geography, many studies using various accessibility indices have been conducted to provide quantitative estimates of the spatial mismatch between supply and demand for these services.

Below, we consider four methods of varying difficulty (see Methods A–D below). The total population of a district is used to represent demand for fresh food, but this can be calculated by replacing population with the number of elderly adults according to one's purpose. Here, the distance within which consumers can access stores without inconvenience is about 10 min on foot or about 500 m distance. In other words, areas with no fresh food store within 500 m are considered to have low food access. It is necessary to change the distance flexibly according to the purpose of the analysis.

Method A: Simple Method Using Map and Pen

The simplest way to estimate supply and demand is using a map and pen. Currently, it is possible to obtain and print seamless digital maps—such as Google Maps—from the Internet. First, print a map of the area to be analyzed and mark the locations of fresh food stores. Then, referring to the scale of the map, draw a circle with a radius of 500 m around each store using a compass. Areas beyond the range of those circles can be regarded as having low food access (Fig. 3.1). In addition, if small-area population data are used, the approximate population of the FDs can also be estimated. In each small area, calculate the percentage of the area outside the circle. Then, by multiplying the proportion of the area outside the circle by the population, it is possible to estimate the population of people with limited access to shopping facilities. For example, in a district where 100 people live, if 60% of the area is not included in the circle, it can be estimated that 60 people have limited access to shopping facilities.

Method B: Method to Compare Census of Commerce Data and Population Data Based on an Area-Wide Mesh (i.e. Grid Square)

Although Method A is highly accurate, it is difficult to confirm all shops' addresses individually on macro scales such as cities and nations. To measure food access on a macro scale, we should use grid-square (area-wide mesh) data from *Commercial Statistics*. In short, one must distinguish whether each mesh is a poor food access area by checking for grocery shops. *Population Census* provides the population data for area-wide meshes. Therefore, it is possible to calculate the population of poor food access meshes.

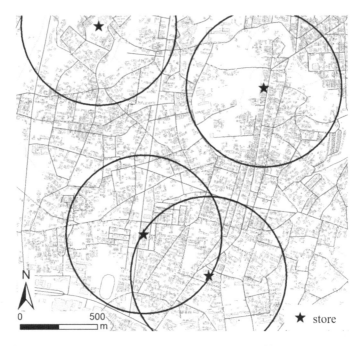

Fig. 3.1 500-meter buffered areas from stores. *Source* Iwama ed. (2017)

However, *Commercial Statistics* does not show the detailed addresses of grocery shops. If a grocery shop is located on the border of an area-wide mesh, the residents of adjacent meshes may also use it. To produce a more accurate food access map, we should consider the presence/absence of grocery stores located in adjacent meshes.

The Research Institute of the Agriculture, Forestry and Fisheries Ministry has developed this idea and made a more accurate and sophisticated food access map (we mention this in an additional note in Sect. 3.2). This map considers both grocery shops inside the mesh as well as those located in adjacent meshes. This institute also estimates the distributions of residents and grocery stores inside a mesh probabilistically and calculates food access accurately.

Method C: Method Based on Road Distance

This section explains the method using the GIS spatial analysis tool. In Method A, distance to a store was measured as a straight 500 m line. However, because people walk along roads, a more precise distance to the store must be measured by road distance. This is not easy to calculate manually, but the 500 m zone in terms of road distance can be derived more easily using GIS. First, it is necessary to prepare point data for each store and line data for digital roads. Using a network analysis tool for

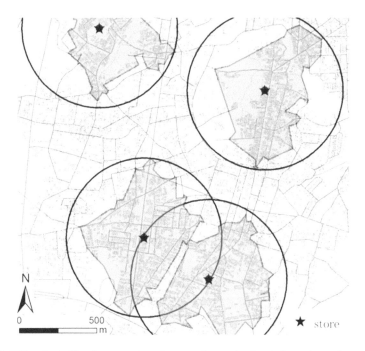

Fig. 3.2 500-meter buffered areas and service areas by road network from stores. *Source* Iwama ed. (2017)

GIS, it is possible to instantly calculate 500 m road distances from each store. As shown in Fig. 3.2, the colored part in the circle is the 500 m zone based on road distance, which is quite different from the 500 m zone calculated by straight line radius. If there are barriers such as rivers and cliffs nearby, large differences are likely in the 500 m area.

Numbers of people with limited access to shopping facilities can be estimated according to the proportion of the area excluded from the 500 m area within each small area, as in Method A. Using GIS allows the population to be estimated more accurately.

Method D: Method Using Kernel Density Estimation (Poor Food Access Map)

Next, we introduce a method to determine areas at high risk for FDs using the kernel density estimation method in GIS. By utilizing regional statistical data, it is possible to identify high-risk areas for FDs according to geographical factors. The kernel density estimation method can measure the surfaces (i.e. density) of supply and those of demand (Silverman 1986).

Figure 3.3 shows a simple example. First, a supply surface representing the food supply density is created from store distributions. As the number of stores and store

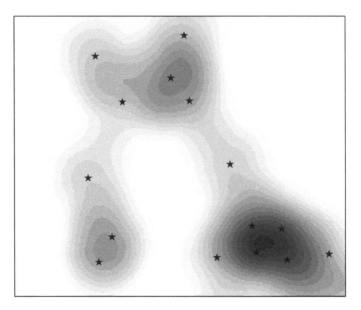

Fig. 3.3 Density surface derived from point distribution. *Source* Iwama ed. (2017)

sizes increase, the supply density increases. In places where density is high, residents have a large supply of fresh food. Similarly, a demand surface can be created from the population distribution.

When we overlay these two surfaces, some areas may show a mismatch; a location where demand far surpasses supply must be an FD area. A place where the demand volume is much higher than the supply volume indicates a shortage of food supply, where many have limited access to shopping facilities.

The kernel density estimator $V(i)$ is found using the equations:

$$V(i) = \sum_{i=1}^{n} K_{ij} \tag{1}$$

$$K_{ij} = \begin{cases} 0 & d_{ij}/h > 1 \\ 3\pi^{-1}\left(1 - d_{ij}/h\right)^2 g_j & d_{ij}/h \le 1 \end{cases} \tag{2}$$

where d_{ij} is the distance between point i and point j, g_j is the weight at point j, and h is a smoothing parameter (or bandwidth). The density at point i is a summation of all g_j within point i to a distance of h. However, weights become lighter with distance from point i.

To estimate the food supply density, j is the grocery store and g_j is the size of the store (e.g. floor space). On the other hand, to calculate the density of food demand, j is the measurement point and g_j is the population. Parameter h is 500 m, which is the critical travel distance to grocery stores.

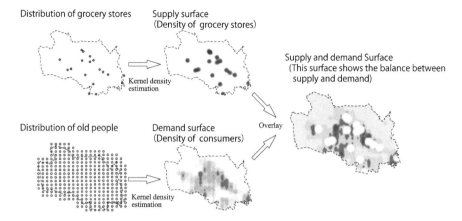

Fig. 3.4 Image of making s poor food access map by kernel density estimation. *Source* Iwama ed. (2017)

In addition, for GIS analysis, it is necessary to create spatial data for stores and populations using various spatial statistics. For grocery stores, a database listing attributes such as store name, address, and sales floor area must be constructed. The latitude and longitude of each store are acquired by geocoding, and point data for the store are created. On the other hand, for the population in relation to demand, we use population data in units of small areas or grids. Population data are converted into point data for their centroid.

An image used for analysis is shown in Fig. 3.4. First, a supply surface is created from a fresh food store using kernel density estimation. Similarly, a demand surface is created from point data on elderly adults. These two surfaces are then overlaid to create a surface that shows the balance between supply and demand. On a surface created in this way, it can be said that the areas where the demand is much higher than supply are at high risk of FDs. We call this a 'poor food access map'.

In many studies, the supply surface is usually created by the stores' total area (m^2), and the demand surface is based on residential population (i.e. people). The fundamental units of these surfaces are different. Therefore, it is impossible to compare them in a simple manner, and many preceding studies only measured the relative balance of demand and supply (Tanaka et al. 2007). To overcome this problem, we create a new supply surface based on the total population of shoppers for all stores (i.e. people). In our research, both surfaces have the base unit of 'population', so we can compare the surfaces directly. To calculate the population of shoppers, we used the calculation method that Large-Scale Retail Store Location Low shows in its guiding principles.[1]

3.2.2   Comparison of Maps Created by Different Methods

3.2.2.1   Four Methods

In the preceding section, we introduced four methods for calculating food access (Methods A–D, mentioned in 3.2.1.2). Are there any differences between the results from these calculation methods? To what extent do the results differ? To answer these questions, we consider the analyses we performed in 2012. We calculated accessibility of stores and estimated the number of disadvantaged shoppers (i.e. those whose house is more than 500 m from the nearest grocery store) using the four methods in the same district. The case study district was X Ward in Tokyo. This district has a variety of residential areas including expensive high-rise apartments for high-income residents, low-rise dwellings for relatively low-income residents, and an old public housing complex where many of the residents are over age 65 years. To compare the four methods statistically, we used GIS.

For the supply surface, we chose stores that satisfied the following conditions: (1) are listed in the *Japan Supermarket Dictionary 2012*, (2) are in X district or within 500 m of its boundary, and (3) sell fresh vegetables. For the demand surface, we used area-wide mesh data on the elderly adult population. As of September 2012, the most recent mesh data (500 m mesh data from the *2010 Population Census*) had not yet been published. Therefore, we used the *2005 Population Census.*[2] These data are published by town and street units. We re-aggregated these data into 500 m mesh units in proportion to the area and set the maximum travel distance for elderly adults at 500 m.

Distance Methods (Buffering) [Methods A and C]

Table 3.1 shows the results derived by each of the four methods (direct distance, road distance, area-wide mesh, and kernel density estimation). Methods A and C, described above, correspond to direct and road distances, respectively. Figure 3.5 shows 500 m buffers (500 m zones around each store) based on direct and road distances. Regarding buffering based on the direct distance, almost all areas of X Ward are within 500 m and only 8.7% are outside this zone. The population living outside this zone numbers 2,852 (4.7%). However, 24.7% of X Ward are outside the 500 m zone calculated based on road distance (network buffering). The population of these poor food access areas is 11,935 (19.7%) (Fig. 3.5).

Table 3.1 Results derived by the four methods

Method	Poor food access areas		Population of disadvantaged shoppers	
	(km²)	(%)	(person)	(%)
Distance methods (buffering)				
direct distance [Method A]	1.6	8.7	2,852	4.7
road distance [Method C]	4.5	24.7	11,935	19.7
Area-wide mesh (grid square) method [Method B]				
500 m grid square	12.3	47.0	33,401	40.3
Kernel density estimation method (poor food access map) [Method D]				
demand>supply	16.0	87.4	54,638	90.2
> average	9.8	53.8	38,633	63.8
> average+1standard deviation	2.3	12.5	10,572	17.5

Source Iwama ed. (2017)

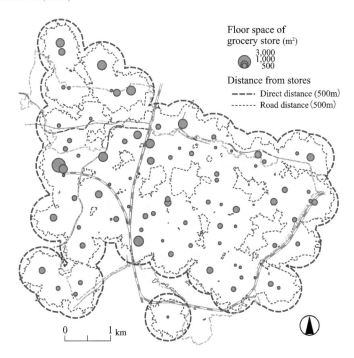

Fig. 3.5 500 m buffers based on direct distance and road distance. *Source* Iwama ed. (2017)

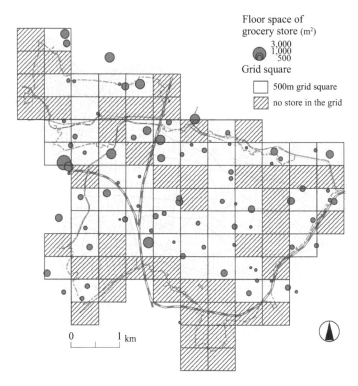

Fig. 3.6 Overlay of supply area and demand area (500 m grid square). *Source* Iwama ed. (2017)

Area-Wide Mesh (Grid Square) Method [Method B]

Method B is based on an area-wide mesh. In Sect. 1.2, we used mesh data to create a supply surface. We obtained store information from the *Commercial Statistics*. However, to compare the four methods, we must homogenize statistical data. Therefore, in this section, we used 500 m area-wide mesh data and distinguished whether each mesh is a poor food access area by checking for grocery stores. We then calculated food accessibility.

Figure 3.6 shows the overlay of the supply area and demand area (500 m grid square). There are 100 mesh areas in X Ward, of which 47 (47.0% of the total population) have no grocery store. The population of these mesh areas is 33,401 (40.3%).

Kernel Density Estimation Method (Poor Food Access Map) [Method D]

The kernel density estimation method corresponds to Method D, and Fig. 3.7 shows the results of demand–supply balance. The average demand–supply balance value is 1,665.7 with a standard deviation of 1,955.3. The proportion of areas where the

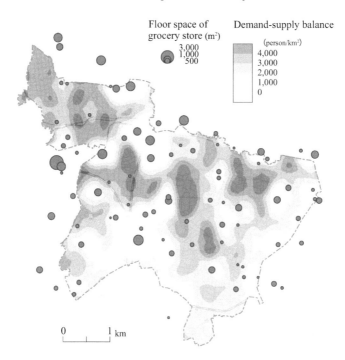

Fig. 3.7 Demand–supply balance by kernel density estimation (poor food access map). *Source* Iwama ed. (2017)

demand surface exceeded the supply surface is 16.0%, with a population of 56,638 (90.2%). In addition, the proportion of areas where the demand–supply balance exceeded the average is 9.8% with a population of 38,633 (63.8%). The ratio of areas where the balance exceeded the average by more than one standard deviation is 2.3% with a population of 10,572 (17.5%).

Comparison of the Four Methods

Table 3.1 suggests that the four methods (Methods A and C, Method B, and Method D) yield different size estimates of poor food access areas and different numbers of disadvantaged shoppers. The largest poor food access areas were calculated by Method D, based on a demand–supply balance value greater than 0 (demand value ≥ supply value). The smallest area sizes and populations were calculated using Method C, based on direct distance. The discrepancy between the result derived from Methods D and C (largest and smallest estimates, respectively) is almost 10 times for area and 19 times for population.

In addition, the method using road distance yielded measures of poor food access areas that were 0.35 times the size of the estimate from the area-based method, and 0.24 times the size of the population estimate from the direct distance method. These gaps occurred because of the road networks in the study area. In X Ward, water areas such as rivers, moats, and public areas including train stations and parks affect road distance.

Moreover, the area-wide mesh method shows wider poor food access areas and a larger population of disadvantaged shoppers than other methods. We suggest the reasons for this discrepancy are: (1) mesh areas were set automatically, so many were unexpectedly classified as 'poor food access areas'; and (2) this analysis extracted many no-grocery-store meshes. However, if the adjacent mesh has a grocery store, the shopping environment and food access of the no-grocery-store meshes must be better than this method predicts.

The above analysis suggests two points: (1) the different methods yield varying results, and (2) local attributes such as road networks, topography, distributions of stores, and statistical units change the results in relation to food access.

These methods use widely available data that cover the whole nation, so it is possible for many people to make FD maps of any locality. In addition, these data may be updated periodically. Therefore, poor food access maps can also be updated. Moreover, mesh data methods are unaffected by changes in administrative districts (i.e. changes in boundaries resulting from the merging of municipalities). We can analyze changes in poor food access areas over time and compare food access areas across cities.

3.2.3   Summary—Toward the Utilization of Food Access Maps

Food access maps are superior for showing where and how large-scale FD issues may arise. Food access maps are also important indices for addressing FDs (through countermeasures) including determining places to open new stores and food delivery services and mobile vending vehicle routes. Furthermore, we can publish food access maps widely via web GIS. If access maps are shared widely, we can easily learn who lives in FD districts (i.e. elderly adult neighbors and relatives). Such information would allow neighbors and relatives to visit these individuals frequently to offer assistance. This grassroots support may be an effective measure by which to address the FD issue.

However, food access mapping is not a panacea. These maps are created based on distance alone, without consideration of other factors. They should not be understood to suggest that all residents of poor food access areas suffer from FDs. Poor food access maps just show the potential areas for FDs. For example, even if the nearest grocery store is located 3 km from a home, families with private cars and those who are affluent enough to order frequent food deliveries would not experience any serious difficulty with living in poor food access areas. On the other hand, even if the nearest grocery store is within 1 km, areas inhabited by many elderly individuals who cannot use private cars likely represent an FD problem. In addition, areas where residents maintain good communication with each other seldom have FD issues. In contrast, even if there are many grocery stores nearby, elderly adults with economic or health difficulties, or those who are isolated from society and stay at home all day, have a high FD risk. In short, to judge whether a research area is an FD, we must focus not only on special accessibility to the stores but also on the existence/absence of a way to overcome distance; moreover, we must focus on the neighborhood community. Food access maps should be used as hazard maps that show possible FDs.[3]

Additional note: The introduction of web maps related to FDs

Recently, government workers and researchers have sought to understand FDs (disadvantaged shoppers) statistically. On this note, we introduce Japanese and US web maps to estimate the number and distribution of FD victims.

1. **Food access map (Policy Research Institute, Ministry of Agriculture, Forestry and Fisheries)** [http://cse.primaff.affrc.go.jp/katsuyat/]

This map is based on an area-wide mesh (half grid square data: 500 m square) covering all of Japan. This map shows the population ratio of people whose homes are more than 500 m from the nearest grocery store. This map is provided in .kml and .pdf formats. We can see .kml-formatted maps from Google Earth against the background of aerial photographs and other data. In addition, by changing the format, we can use this map with other GIS software. This map uses permanent populations listed in the *2010 Population Census*, and the number of grocery stores listed in *Commercial Statistics 2007* to estimate food access in each mesh. This map corresponds to results from Method B, the area-wide mesh method mentioned in Sect. 3.2. However, this poor food access map adapts a stochastic model[4] to maximize its precision. This map uses many techniques, such as estimating store locations in each mesh by probability theory and controlling for the effects of stores located in adjacent meshes. It estimates that the number of disadvantaged shoppers is 4.6 million (including 1.1 million individuals over the age of 65 years).

There is a degree of error between the estimates of the food access map and the actual town street-level situations. However, the estimations at the municipality level (city and prefecture levels) are sufficiently accurate. This map clearly shows the distribution of potential FD areas from food access viewpoints. This map is expected to be used by municipalities to remedy FDs or by food retailers for area marketing. This website also introduces the report from this project (in .pdf format). This report shows the proportion of the population who are disadvantaged shoppers and their areas of distribution. This report also introduces another food access map that considers the distribution of convenience stores.

2. **Food Desert Locator (United States Department of Agriculture)** [http://www.ers.usda.gov/data-products/food-access-research-atlas/go-to-the-atlas.aspx]

The United States Department of Agriculture (USDA) has announced the census tracts classified as FDs. On these tracts, we can see detailed information about the total population, the population of elderly adults, low-income earners, carless households, and other information. The low-income information is worth mentioning. In Japan, it is impossible to obtain individual-level financial data, although income is one of the most important FD factors. Analyzing these financial data would drastically improve our FD map. The USDA FD maps use a 1 km mesh unit, with the distance from the center point of each mesh to the nearest supermarket (there are 40,108 supermarkets in the USA). In urban areas, being more than 1.6 km (1 mile) from the nearest grocery store is a criterion for a poor food access area. In rural areas, on the other hand, the index distance is more than 16 km. This website defines an FD as a census tract: (1) where the total population of residents who live in poor food access areas is more than 500, or (2) where more than one-third of residents live in poor food access areas. As a result, about 6,529 tracts are defined as FDs and about 1.36 million residents (52.8% of the total population of these tracts) are estimated to be victims of FD issues.

3.   **Procedure for measuring social capital from the viewpoint of health**

In Sect. 3.3, we introduce the measurement procedure for social capital (SC) from the viewpoint of health.

3.2.4   What Is Social Capital?

I was born and raised in a city on the outskirts of Tokyo where neighbors maintain good relationships. As a child, they treated me well; neighborhood adults were kind, local children were good friends, and we were remarkably close. If someone had serious problems, we often noticed it soon and helped them. Sharing meals was common. Middle-aged women (i.e. of my grandmother's and mother's generations) often chatted on side streets and enjoyed gossiping beside the well. If outsiders came into our neighborhood, we noticed them. My neighborhood was safe enough for us to leave the entrance door unlocked when we went out.

During my childhood, I thought that such close neighborhood communities were common. However, after I left my parents' house, I realized that such friendly communities are rare. There was no intimate neighborhood in the student quarters of my university, nor were there intimate neighborhoods in the residential areas where I lived after graduating. In 2015, I lived alone in Edinburgh, UK, for a year. My English was not good, and I only stayed for a short time, so I could not form close relationships with my neighbors there. When I came back to my flat at night, I sometimes felt lonely. No one shared meals with me. I did not even know who my neighbors were. This was a so-called high-end residential area with good security. However, when I went out, I triple locked my door. (Now I really like the UK and I strongly hope to return there soon.) When I had trouble there, I asked my friends living in other districts or my university colleagues for help, not my neighbors. When I arrived in the UK, I had no acquaintances there and was completely isolated. When I was a child, my neighborhood maintained high SC and we lived in peace. On the other hand, I did not find my UK neighborhood to be a close community. If people are isolated from society, even if they are young and in good health, they feel uneasy.

SC refers to social networks (i.e. ties with people and groups) and normative consciousness based on trust and reciprocity (Putnam 2000). If people or groups believe in each other, have sufficiently good relationships and help each other, and communicate positively and regularly, they can feel a sense of security. When they have problems, they can cooperate to help each other and overcome them. These social networks are called SC. If people trust, help, and have daily contact with others, neighbors often become cooperative.

SC is especially important for elderly adults. In general, as people age, they selectively lose their ties with others. Typical cases are the ties with a Parent–Teacher Association and the workplace. If their children graduate from school, the parents' community will dissolve. Likewise, even if people have a wide range of relationships at work, they lose many of these after retirement. Family members and friends are similar. Children leave their parents' homes sooner or later. Some friends will die eventually. In addition, as they age (and decrease in strength), it becomes difficult for elderly adults to maintain relationships with their friends from far-away places at the same level as in their youth. On the other hand, emotional intimacy with a few close friends increases. In addition, the feeling of social embeddedness is enhanced (Koyano and Ando 2008). Elderly adults' range of activities thus become reduced. Consequently, neighbors are particularly important for elderly adults to retain social ties.

The neighbors in my hometown are also aging now. On the side streets, the same people (now over age 65 years) still enjoy chatting. My aunt, who lives in the same city, frequently comes to my parents' home and goes shopping with my mother. An elderly gentleman, who was busy until he retired, is now always in his garden, growing plants and washing his car. He also enjoys chatting with neighbors when they pass by his garden. This gentleman is now a key member of the community. An elderly woman who was always affectionate when I was a child is in poor health and rarely goes shopping by herself. However, the neighbors (especially the elderly gentleman) always support her. The neighbors, including my parents, really like this community. My mother often tells me that 'I would not move away from here even if my husband passed away and I became single'. It is safe to say that these neighborhood communities (and their social relationships) provide especially important SC.

3.2.5 The Fear of a 'Muen-Shakai' (Isolated Society)

If SC is lost, desolation will expand widely in society. In 2010, Nippon Hosou Kyokai (NHK: the Japan Broadcasting Corporation) broadcast a documentary program titled *'Muen-Shakai'* (isolated society). This program deeply shocked Japanese society.[5] The word 'Muen-Shakai' was coined by the mass media to mean a society where residents lose social ties with one another and family, becoming isolated from society. According to this program, there are 32,000 who contracted disease or died on journey (i.e. the person or body is unidentifiable and unclaimed). When the government finds a person who contracted disease or died on journey, it releases a short description of the person's information, including height, weight, and belongings in its official gazette. This small article is all the available information about the person. This TV program focused on one who contracted disease or died on journey and investigated his life history based on several clues. It was difficult to discover his history because few people knew him. Finally, this program revealed the person's life history. He was an average person who was born and grew up in a small town. He found a job and was married in his hometown. He worked hard but unfortunately his company went bankrupt. Then he moved to Tokyo. At that time, he was divorced from his wife. In Tokyo, he also worked hard and had friends at work. However, after his retirement at age 60, he gradually became isolated from society. Eventually, he led a lonely life and died alone in his cheap apartment. There was little communication among the residents of his apartment building, and no one noticed his death for more than a week after he died. This TV program taught us that isolation from society is not something unrelated to us. Moreover, this program sounded the alarm on *Muen-Shakai*.

Our research team studied an elderly housing complex in Tokyo a few years ago. This large-scale housing complex was built in the 1960s and many of its residents are now over 65 years old (Photo 3.1). More than 20,000 elderly adults live there. The neighborhood relationships are very weak in this housing complex. Although

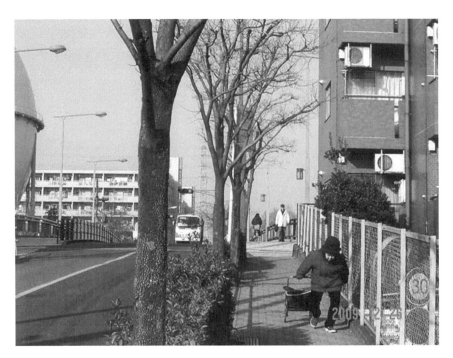

Photo 3.1   The elderly person in the large-scale housing complex (Itabashi Ward, 2009, taken by Iwama)

many residents have lived there for several decades, few people know their neighbors well. Some members of neighborhood associations and nonprofit organizations have attempted to build a neighborhood community. They hold neighborhood meetings regularly and have established clubs, such as sports clubs and cultural clubs, but few people are interested in these activities. We received full support from this neighborhood association and conducted a questionnaire survey about residents' living environments. As expected, their social ties were very weak. We found that many residents had unhealthy eating habits. We were surprised at the responses that residents wrote in the free spaces of our questionnaire sheets. They declared their loneliness and anxieties with phrases such as 'I feel lonely', 'I am really afraid of nighttime', 'I used to live in this room with many family members, but now I am alone', and 'my neighbor does not seem to have gone out for many months. She is very old. I worry about her'. Of course, some residents live with their families and neighbors and enjoy their lives in this complex. However, it is also true that many people are isolated from society and live alone in their small room. Through this research, we glimpsed the actual state of *Muen-Shakai*. SC i s at least as important to our living environment as social infrastructure such as grocery stores and public transportation.

3.2.6 Relationship Between Local Social Capital and Health

SC is used as a research construct in many fields because it is a useful tool for gaining a comprehensive understanding of issues related to families and local communities (Kawachi et al. 1997; Kawachi et al. 2008; Kondo 2007). However, there is a lack of consensus about SC analyses. Moreover, agreement on the definition of the concept, measurement methodology, and causal relationships remain elusive, with approaches differing according to academic discipline.

Research on SC and health has been concentrated in fields such as social epidemiology, public health, and dietetics.[6] The relationships between SC and health disturbances have been academically proven; mortality (Martikainen et al. 2003), self-rated health (Kawachi et al. 1999; Kim et al. 2006a), mental health (Fujiwara and Kawachi 2008; Lofors and Sundquist 2007), and health behaviors (Kim et al. 2006b; Poortinga 2006) have all been related to SC. The routes by which SC influences health have been broadly divided between the individual and local levels. Many studies have empirically demonstrated that ties at the individual level (i.e. interactions with family, friends and/or acquaintances) and the mutual aid created in those interactions have a major influence on people's health maintenance (Kawachi 1997). However, in recent years, there has been increasing interest in the influence of locality on residents' health status (i.e. their ties with social organizations and with the community) (Lindström et al. 2002; Subramanian and Duncan 2003; Kondo 2007, Nakaya and Hanibuchi 2013). In other words, is it possible that local ties—not just individual ties—contribute to residents' health maintenance? One could also ask whether individuals with no social ties at the individual level can enjoy a certain level of benefits simply by living in a community that is rich in SC. Some social epidemiologists say 'yes', showing examples of aggressive approaches by members of the Consumer Affairs Committee to help isolated elderly adults.[7] The Japanese government appoints a representative of each town street to be a member of the Consumer Affairs Committee. If members of the Consumer Affairs Committee are cordial in their approach to isolated elderly adults, they create healthy, trusting relationships. These elderly adults may participate in local activities such as neighborhood dinner parties. Even if the elderly individual rejects these approaches, members of the Consumer Affairs Committee will contact public health nurses and inform them of the elderly individual's condition. Then the public health nurses will contact the elderly adults and take care of them.

It is easy for me to imagine that local SC may contribute to residents' health maintenance. As mentioned above, my hometown has high local-level SC. If elderly individuals moved to this street, many residents, including the elderly gentleman I mentioned above, may approach the newcomers and invite them into the neighborhood community. If such elderly adults had poor eating habits, the gentleman would treat them to his signature seafood dishes, which he catches and cooks himself. FD issues seldom arise in such communities.

3.2.7 Measurement Method for SC: Measuring Respondents' Interactions with Neighbors

SC is a particularly important concept in FD studies. How can we measure local SC? In this and the next section, we introduce two measurement methods. The first method is relatively easy. This method can measure research subjects' interactions with their neighbors using a questionnaire survey (Asakawa 2005). There are nine levels of choices from '1. Do you say "hello" to your neighbors?' to '9. Do you go on overnight trips with your neighbors?'(Table 3.2). These choices are directly proportional to the intimacy with neighbors ('choice 1' is the most distant relationship and 'choice 9' is the closest). Specifically, we ask research subjects to imagine their neighbors who live to the right of their residence and answer the above questions with 'yes' or 'no'. If subjects answer 'no' to '1. Do you say "hello" to your neighbors?', that means their relationship is too weak. In contrast, if they answer 'yes' to '8. Do you lend things (such as seasonings like salt and sugar) to, and borrow things from, your neighbors?' or '9. Do you go on overnight trips with your neighbors?', then their relationship is very strong.

In our case study of the housing complexes I mentioned above, 90.0% of respondents answered 'yes' to '1. Do you say "hello" to your neighbors',[8] but only 76.6% answered 'yes' to '2. Do you know your neighbor's family structure?' and 48.3% answered 'yes' to '3. Do know your neighbor's occupation?'. We speculate that many residents prefer individualism and have an unspoken code of conduct to keep each other at a distance and not invade each other's privacy.[9]

Table 3.2 Respondents' interactions with their neighbors (the ratio of 'yes' responses)

	Total (%)	Male (%)	Female (%)
say hello to their neighbors	90.0	91.8	89.1
visit their neighbors houses or invite neighbors to their house*	76.6	64.4	83.6
know their neighbor's family construction	48.3	42.5	51.6
know their neighbor householder's occupation*	43.4	31.9	50.0
gave souvenirs to neighbors or get souvenirs from their neighbors*	24.9	16.4	29.7
talk to their neighbors about their concerns*	21.9	9.6	28.9
borrow something (i.e. seasonings such as soy source) from their neighbors or lend something to neighbors	14.6	8.2	18.3
go out with their neighbors*	11.6	4.1	15.9
go on a journey with their neighbors	2.5	1.4	3.2

Note ** $p < .01$, * $p < .05$
Source Iwama et al. (2011), Iwama ed. (2017)

However, some residents maintain a moderate relationship with neighbors, as exemplified by 'I know my neighbor's family structure'. We proved statistically that this moderate relationship might prevent residents from being isolated. Moreover, our study showed that neighbors who maintain moderate relationships tend to have healthy eating habits (Iwama 2013). On the other hand, many elderly adults who 'do not know their neighbor's family structure' are isolated from their neighbors and family members. These people's daily eating habits are generally bad. We found the same tendency in other research areas. Many urban people do not like close relationships with neighbors, whereas close relationships are common in rural areas. Maintaining close relationships with neighbors is often difficult in urban areas. Our research suggests that even if we do not maintain close relationships with neighbors, moderate ties with neighbors may prevent us from being isolated and falling into poor eating habits. It is safe to say that '2. Do you know your neighbor's family structure?' is a key indicator of the risk of isolation from the neighborhood.

This method is simple. We can easily measure the risk of isolation from the neighborhood using this method. However, SC has a complicated structure. This method can only measure structural SC but cannot be used to analyze cognitive SC (which we mention below). To understand SC well, we must research it comprehensively.

3.2.8   Measurement Method for SC: Comprehensive Measurement

SC is measured using a variety of indicators. Table 3.3 shows the main indicators of the relationship between SC and the health of elderly individuals (Kondo 2014;

Table 3.3 Main indicators of the relationship between SC and elderly people's health

Main indicators		Example
1.	Participation in social organizations with a vertical social structure	Neighborhood associations or clubs for the elderly
2.	Participation in social organizations with a horizontal social structure	Volunteer groups, sports clubs, or hobby clubs
3.	Level of relationships with neighbors	Exchanging greetings, borrowing things, or getting together for meals
4.	Breadth of relationships with neighbors	Frequency of interaction or number of people
5.	Feelings of trust	Whether they trust people and society
6.	Reciprocity norms	Whether they are motivated to participate in local events such as festivals or volunteering

Source Kondo (2014) [partly revised], Iwama ed. (2017)

Berkman and Kawachi 2000): (1) participation in social organizations with a vertical social structure, (2) participation in social organizations with a horizontal social structure, (3) level of relationships with neighbors, (4) breadth of relationships with neighbors, (5) feelings of trust, and (6) reciprocity norms.

Among these, indicators (1)–(4) are denoted as structural SC, which pertains to social relationships and is indicative of people's roles in social groups and network membership. Indicators (5) and (6) correspond to cognitive SC, which is the norms, values, and beliefs of social group members. Cognitive SC provides the foundation for structural SC and is reinforced by structural SC in a mutually complementary relationship.

Because cognitive SC pertains to individuals, influencing it via external means is difficult. Yet because structural SC has a strong social dimension, a certain amount of improvement can be expected from initiatives such as creating opportunities for social participation or establishing centers for social interaction. Thus, researchers studying the relationship between health and SC frequently examine and diagnose problems in the local community based on structural SC and provide local feedback based on the results. We share this perspective.

Large amounts of quantitative data are needed to empirically analyze the relationship between an individual's health status (the dependent variable) and SC (the independent variable). However, there are limits regarding the data that can be used, because health status and SC involve individual privacy. Moreover, standard measures of the relationship between health status and SC have yet to be developed.

To date, in case studies of Japanese seniors, the principal indicators that have been verified as having statistically significant relationships are: self-rated health (dependent) and sense of trust (independent); certification rate of the need for long-term care (dependent) and participation in horizontal social organizations (independent); rate of falls (dependent) and participation in horizontal social organizations (independent); number of remaining teeth (dependent) and extent/number of relationships with neighbors (independent); depression (dependent) and participation in horizontal social organizations (independent); self-rated health and self-rated happiness (dependent) and the SC indicators of sense of trust, reciprocity norms, and participation in horizontal social organizations (independent) (Kondo 2007).

Although the current study builds on a series of studies relating to SC and health status, the wide array of SC indicators that have been used makes it difficult to develop a comprehensive explanation of how health is affected by SC. However, the presence or absence of ties with family and the local community directly influences the problem of FDs. These ties can be expected to be sources of support for a person's daily living (i.e. people shopping on another person's behalf, sharing things they have been given, or inviting the person for a meal in a group). Thus, for the analysis in this study, ties with family and the local community were included as indicators. Specifically, these ties were measured quantitatively using 'frequency of participation in local clubs and events' and 'the presence of someone to eat meals with or the frequency of meals in groups'.

SC is a complicated concept and measuring it is difficult. Recently, some papers and books have proposed measures of SC (Kondo 2007, 2014; Nakaya and Hanibuchi 2013). Kondo (2007) proposed the questionnaire used in his research and, after pointing out that no clear SC measurement index yet exists, showed some provisional research indices (Kondo 2014).

In this book, we used several methods to measure SC in central Tokyo, a prefectural government city, and a small town (for more detail, please see Chapters 4–6).

3.2.9 Summary—SC Research Considerations

It is quite difficult to measure SC on a macro scale, such as within town streets and cities. Nevertheless, we received full support from the government to conduct a large-scale survey. We proceeded with the survey in cooperation with interdisciplinary researchers such as sociologists, statisticians, nutritionists, and epidemiologists. In addition, we received research funds from the Japanese government. Full government support, a wide range of interdisciplinary knowledge, and a certain amount of research funds are necessary to conduct SC research.

Research indices and evaluation criteria are unclear in SC measurement. These technical issues also make SC research difficult. In the case of shopping activities, many academic research studies show that elderly adults can walk for an average of 1 km.[10] Therefore, it is safe to say that if the distance between home and the nearest grocery store is over 500 m (1 km there and back), it is difficult for an elderly individual to go shopping without a car. Therefore, we can make a food access map with the distance between home and the nearest grocery store (index) and a 500 m distance (limit value). On the other hand, in the case of SC, index and limit value are unclear at this stage. To make a n SC map, we should accumulate more SC studies.

Recently, the Japan Agency for Gerontology Evaluation Study (JAGES)[11] has conducted large-scale surveys of the entire nation on a regular basis to ascertain the health conditions and SC of elderly Japanese adults. It is also making a data platform and sharing its data with many interdisciplinary researchers. Its project makes it easier for researchers to investigate SC comprehensively. We expect that this project will soon create established indices and limit values with which to measure local SC.

3.3   Conclusions

In this chapter, we have introduced how to measure food access and local SC. Recently, many researchers have been analyzing the indices of food access and SC. We have introduced some that are highly practical. These analyses have continued. We hope new and more useful indices will be developed soon. It is already possible to create FD maps. Therefore, in the following chapters, we explain the FD issues empirically in the central districts of Tokyo, a prefectural capital city, and a small city, creating FD research maps of each.

Notes

1. In municipalities with populations of less than 400,000, the number of shoppers can be calculated using the formula: S_j means floor space (m^2) of store
$$jC_j = \begin{array}{ll} 1100 - 0.03 \times \frac{S_j}{1000} & S_j < 5000 \\ 0.95 \times S_j & S_j \geq 5000 \end{array}.$$
2. https://www.e-stat.go.jp/gis. Accessed 20 July 2020.
3. Nagano Prefecture also researched the shopping environment of prefectural inhabitants over age 65 years and the implementation of disadvantaged shopper services.
4. For more detail, see (Yakushiji and Takahashi 2012).
5. This TV programme was published as a book (NHK 2010).
6. For more detail, see (Kondo 2007).
7. For more detail, see (Kondo 2014).
8. These data are based on a questionnaire survey. Generally, the response rate by active individuals is higher than among those who are inactive. Therefore, these data appear more positive than the community may actually be. A member of this area's self-government society suggested that the proportion of those who say 'hello' to their neighbors is less than 50%.
9. Some residents responded that they do not like the local community and intentionally refuse to communicate with neighbors.
10. It is expected that in the three major metropolitan areas (Tokyo, Osaka, and Nagoya), it is difficult for 51% of elderly adults aged 65–74 years and 77% of those over 75 years to walk further than 1 km alone. In small towns, it is difficult for 53% of elderly adults aged 65–74 years and 80% of those over 75 years to walk further than 1 km alone. http://www.mlit.go.jp/common/001087037.pdf#search='%E9%83%BD%E5%B8%82%E3%81%AB%E3%81%8A%E3%81%91%E3%82%8B%E4%BA%BA%E3%81%AE%E5%8B%95%E3%81%8D'. Accessed 20 July 2020.
11. http://www.jages.net/. Accessed 20 July 2020.

References

Asakawa T (2005) Elderly females and society. Health and Active Aging 11:56–77 (Japanese with English abstract)

Berkman L, Kwachi I (2000) Social epidemiology. Oxford University Press, New York

Fujiwara T, Kawachi I (2008) A prospective study of individual-level social capital and major depression in the United States. J Epidemiol Community Health 62(7):627–633

Iwama N (ed) (2013) Revised version. Food desert issues in Japan: Food desert caused by isolated society. Association of Agriculture and Forestry Statistics, Tokyo (Japanese)

Iwama N (ed) (2017) Urban food deserts issues: urban food deserts in low-social capital areas. Association of Agriculture and Forestry Statistics, Tokyo (Japanese)

Kawachi I, Kennedy B, Lochner K, Prothrow SD (1997) Social capital, income inequality, and mortality. Am J Public Health 87(9):1491–1498

Kawachi I, Kennedy BP, Glass R (1999) Social capital and self-rated health: a contextual analysis. Am J Public Health 89(8):1187–1193

Kawachi I, Subramanian SV, Kim D (eds) (2008) Social capital and health. Springer, New York

Kim D, Subramanian SV, Kawachi I (2006a) Bonding versus bridging social capital and their associations with self rated health: a multilevel analysis of 40 US communities. J Epidemiol Community Health 60(2):116–122

Kim D, Subramanian SV, Gortmaker SL, Kawachi I (2006b) US state- and county-level social capital in relation to obesity and physical inactivity: a multilevel, multivariable analysis. Soc Sci Med 63(4):1045–1059

Kondo K (2007) Health disparity society: social epidemiological large research study towards care prevention. Igaku shoin, Tokyo (Japanese)

Kondo K (2014) Social capital and health. In: Inaba Y (ed), Social capital: what is the science of 'the bonds'? (pp 66–96). Miberuba-shobo Ltd, Tokyo (Japanese)

Koyano W, Ando T (2008) Revised edition—new social gerontology: whereabouts of senior life. World Planning Ltd, Tokyo (Japanese)

Lindström M, Merlo J, Ostergren PO (2002) Individual and neighbourhood determinants of social participation and social capital: a multilevel analysis of the city of Malmö. Sweden. Social Science & Medicine 54(2):1797–1805

Lofors J, Sundquist K (2007) Low-linking social capital as a predictor of mental disorders: A cohort study of 4.5 million Swedes. Soc Sci & Med 64(1):21–34

Martikainen P, Kauppinen TM, Valkonen T (2003) Effects of the characteristics of neighbourhoods and the characteristics of people on cause specific mortality: a register based follow up study of 252 000 men. J Epidemiol Community Health 57:210–217

Nakaya T, Hanibuchi T (2013) Neighbourhood inequalities in health and income in Japan. Ann Assoc Econ Geogr 59(1):57–72 (Japanese)

NHK (2010) Muen-Shakai (isolated society): the impact of 32 thousand people who died on journey per year. Bungeishunju, Ltd, Tokyo (Japanese)

Poortinga W (2006) Do health behaviours mediate the association between social capital and health? Prev Med 43(6):488–493

Putnam RD (2000) Bowling alone: the collapse and revival of American community. Simon & Schuster, New York

Silverman BW (1986) Density estimation. Chapman and Hall, London

Subramanian SV, Jones K, Duncan C (2003) Multilevel methods for public health research. In: Kawachi I, Berkman L (eds) Neighborhoods and health. Oxford University Press, New York, pp 65–111

Tanaka K, Iwama N, Sasaki M (2007) Isolation of elderly people and deterioration of living environment in the central part of local city. Daiichi-jutaku-kensetsu-kyokai, Tokyo (Japanese)

Yakushiji T, Takahashi K (2012) Estimation of population classified by distance to the nearest fresh food store: Using grid-square statistics of Population Census and Census of Commerce. Theory and Applications of GIS 20(1):31–37 (Japanese with English abstract)

Part I
The Shopping Environment in Edinburgh, UK

As we mentioned in Chapter 1, studies on the food desert issue started in the UK. Many papers show that the bad eating habits and health hazard issues due to the deterioration of shopping environments in the UK have had many victims, the main of these being low-income people including unskilled workers, single mothers and old people. So, what is the UK's shopping environment? I stayed in the UK from 2014 to 2015. Edinburgh is one of my favourite cities in the UK. Therefore, in this column, I would like to introduce my short-term observation of Edinburgh's shopping environment.

UK's streets are very beautiful (Photo 1). Its shopping streets are full of customers. Unlike Japanese shopping streets, UK's shopping streets are strictly protected by laws which restrict large-scale retailers' activities. Public transportation is advanced, and people can go anywhere in this city using the public bus. However, UK's bicycles are not very useful to old people. Generally, UK uses sport type bicycles and they are permitted to go only on bicycle paths adjacent to a roadway. In Japan, many old people use city cycle type bicycles (speed is slower, but they are easy to pedal

Photo 1 Landscape of Edinburgh 1 (Edinburgh City, 2015, taken by Iwama)

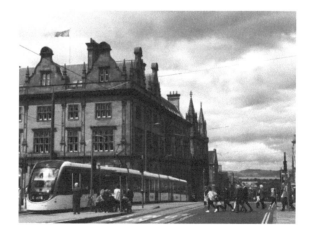

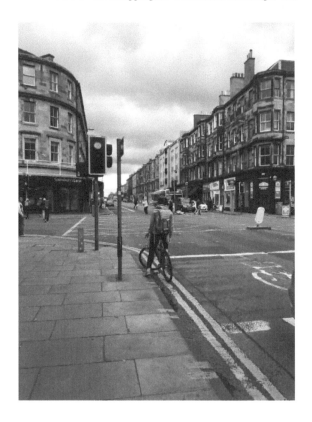

and convenient for carrying heavy luggage) which are designed for everyone's use. Moreover, there are many steep slopes in Edinburgh. So, it seems difficult for an old person to use a bicycle for shopping in this city.

There are various types of grocery stores in Edinburgh. Lots of small and medium size supermarkets are located in this city. These stores are built to harmonize with the surrounding historical landscape (Photo 2). Many stores close by 21:00, but a few stores keep operating until 00:00 or later. Supermarkets are differentiated by their goods' quality and prices. In Edinburgh, we often see supermarket chains such as Sainsbury's and TESCO which are ranked "standard level". These stores' prices of vegetables and meats are almost the same as those of standard supermarkets in Japan. With regard to mutton and beef, which are famous products in Scotland, they are cheaper and of better quality compared with those sold in Japan. Their range of potatoes are also plentiful. In addition, the line-up of retort and frozen foods are abundant. On the other hand, there is a lack in their range of certain fresh foods, especially fresh fish.

There are many low-price supermarkets in Edinburgh. For example, ASDA's suburban type supermarkets are very big and have quite a large range of products such as foods, clothes, commodity goods, etc. Especially, their range of retort and frozen foods deserve a special mention. Customers walk around with large carts and enjoy their shopping. Products' prices are very reasonable. It is safe to say that these stores provide to not only standard customers but also many low-income people. On the other hand, their range of fresh foods seems to be much smaller than that of a Japanese standard supermarket.

Some higher-priced supermarkets like Waitrose are also located in this city. The quality and the price of their goods are much higher than that of other supermarkets. Their range of fresh foods are abundant. We can buy various kinds of fresh meats, fish and vegetables there. The majority of customers at these stores seem to be rich foreigners and from upper-class households.

We can also find many independent corner shops on the streets. These stores sell many kinds of commodity goods, newspapers, lottery tickets, etc. They also sell foods such as a small range of fruits, vegetables, processed meats, eggs and milk. The prices at these shops are relatively higher than those at supermarkets. The managers and staff are generally kind, and the shops have a homely atmosphere. We can enjoy small talk with them.

In addition, we can also see many kinds of specialized stores like butcher shops and fishmongers. Many of them are individual stores. Their floor space may not be large, but the quality is high and the assortment of fresh foods they have in stock is large. They also provide special kinds of meats and fish which we cannot get in supermarkets. They often cut fish and meat on customers' requests (i.e., to fillet the fish). The prices of their fresh foods are relatively high, but these stores have many regular customers.

There are also many kinds of ethnic stores such as Indian, Muslim and Asian shops. They stock various ranges of ethnic foods and products. For example, at Asian stores we can get many kinds of Japanese foods including Japanese soy source, fermented soybean paste (Miso), instant noodles, snacks, etc. Their prices are usually two or three times higher than that in Japan. But many Asians living in this city come and enjoy shopping at these Asian stores. However, even in these stores, Japanese rice is rare and difficult to find. One of the most popular types of rice in Edinburgh is *Yome Nishili* (Photo 3). This rice has a Japanese name but is produced in Europe. The taste of *Yome Nishili* is almost similar to that of Japanese rice. (However, in my opinion, real Japanese rice tastes a little bit better than this European rice).

It is said that it was very difficult to get a wide range of fresh foods in Edinburgh until 10 years ago when the number of resident foreigners began to increase rapidly. There were few ethnic stores until 10 years ago and the assortment of fresh food at the supermarkets was much worse than it is now. Moreover, almost all stores were closed a week before and after Christmas. So, people had to stock rations for two weeks. It seems that the shopping environment of Edinburgh was difficult at that time.

Dining out is expensive in the UK and many people eat meals at home. Basically, they purchase ingredients at grocery stores and cook their own meals. Shopping places generally differ depending on people's social class. The so-called "upper-class" people hardly visit low-price supermarkets, and low-income families do not usually buy their daily foods from expensive stores.

Photo 3 European rice
"Yume nishiki" (Edinburgh
City, 2015, taken by Iwama)

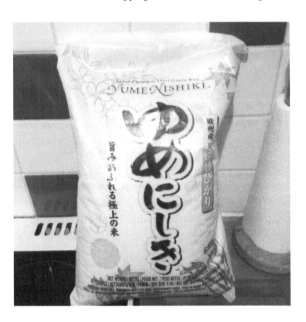

There are also many fast food shops in the town including shops for fish and chips, hamburgers, kebabs and pizzas. Some people eat dinner at these shops, following which they may go to a pub to enjoy a drink.

There are many grocery stores in Edinburgh, so I am sure that few people suffer from an inconvenient shopping environment. However, the issue of poor eating habit in the UK can be as serious as, or more serious than, that in Japan.

Chapter 4
Case Study 1 (Central Tokyo)

Abstract The purposes of this chapter are (1) to verify the existence of urban food deserts in central Tokyo and (2) analyze their characteristics. The case study area is Minato Ward in central Tokyo. The average income of Minato Ward inhabitants is the highest in Japan. Minato Ward is generally considered as a celebrity area free from social exclusion, such as food deserts. Many luxury grocers exist in these districts. However, we found that many elderly residents suffer from high malnutrition risk. This study clarified that personal attributes, such as sex (women) and age, have a statistically significant relationship with healthy eating habits. In addition, the ties with families and neighbors, and family income also have a strong influence on healthy eating. Urban city centers, such as central Tokyo, are at serious risk of urban food desert issues expanding widely among isolated elderly persons.

Keywords Urban food deserts · Celebrity area in central Tokyo · Luxury grocers · Economical gap · Ties with families and neighbors

4.1 Introduction

4.1.1 Characteristics of Food Desert Area in Central Tokyo

The purposes of this chapter are (1) to verify the existence of urban food deserts in central Tokyo and (2) analyze their characteristics. The case study area is Minato Ward, a special ward in Tokyo, Japan. Generally, Minato Ward is considered "a fashionable area." Moreover, Shirokanedai, Azabu, and Roppongi Hills, which are in Minato Ward, have become synonymous with "celebrity residential areas." The average income of Minato Ward inhabitants is the highest in Japan. On the one hand, many of these high-income inhabitants have built up their huge wealth in a single generation. On the other hand, a diverse variety of people also live in this ward, such as the middle-class families who have lived in this district for generations,[1] single professionals, or foreigners. In addition, low-income elderly persons also live in Minato Ward.[2]

Many luxury independent food retailers and supermarkets can be found in Minato Ward; however, for the ward's middle- and low-income residents, these luxury shopping environments might be food poverty areas. Moreover, in areas where residents from various social classes are mixed, it is often difficult to create a local community (social capital) because of the differences in the residents' values and life habits. Residents may often move from their neighborhood to a cheaper area because of the high land rent and inheritance tax, which also hinders the creation of local communities. In short, the risk that the living environment (food access and social capital) in central Tokyo will deteriorate is higher compared with local cities.

Therefore, in this chapter, we discuss the possibility of the existence of food deserts in urban areas. In particular, we analyze the following five points.

1. The creation of food access maps of Tokyo and the introduction of the outline of Minato Ward.
2. The understanding of the diversity of Minato Ward inhabitants and the issue of poverty in elderly persons.
3. Inhabitants' eating habits and their characteristics (District A: a low food access area) [Sects. 4.4.1–4.4.7. Source: Asakawa (2013) and Ishii (2013)].
4. Inhabitants' eating habits and their characteristics (District B: a high food access area) [Sects. 4.5.1–4.5.5. Source: Iwama et al. (2011)].
5. The possibility of the existence of urban food deserts.

Considering point 3, the data were based on the research performed by the Faculty of Sociology and Social Work at Meiji-Gakuin University. These researchers analyzed the relationships between elderly persons' eating behaviors, personal characteristics (e.g., sex, living place, income), and their social networks (e.g., family, friends, acquaintances, neighbors). Considering point 4, the data were based on our research. We also analyzed the relationships between elderly persons' eating behaviors, personal characteristics, and their social networks. The study subjects for points 3 and 4 are basically identical. However, the research areas, question items, and research methods differ slightly between points 3 and 4.

4.1.2   Organization

This chapter comprises four sections. In Sect. 4.2, we discuss the distribution of low food access areas (this section falls within point 1). In Sect. 4.3, we examine the diversity of Minato Ward inhabitants and the issue of poverty in elderly persons (this section falls within point 2). In Sects. 4.4 and 4.5, we introduce the case studies for Districts A and B. District A has few food retailers, while District B has relatively high food access. We analyze the relationship between inhabitants' eating habits and their attributes (this section falls within points 3 and 4). Finally, in Sect. 4.6, we discuss the possibility of the existence of urban food deserts in central Tokyo (this section falls within point 5).

4.1.3 Food Diversity

The investigation of food diversity concerned the frequency of consumption of 10 food groups (meat, fish and shellfish, eggs, milk, processed soy products, green and yellow vegetables, seaweed, fruit, potatoes, and oil and fat) (Kumagai et al. 2003). Respondents were asked to indicate how often they ate each food listed above on the following scale: (1) almost every day; (2) every other day; (3) once or twice a week; or (4) almost never. The number of "almost every day" responses was used as the dietary diversity score. People with low dietary diversity scores (less than 4) have a very high probability of developing poor nutritional health in future. The investigation of food diversity provides a useful index for measuring the healthy eating habits of elderly persons.

Japanese nutrition science has reported that about 80% of Japanese standard meals including main dishes, side dishes are made with the 10 food groups mentioned above. For elderly persons, basic skills are necessary for living independently, including 'Instrumental activities for daily living', 'Intellectual activities', and 'Social role'.[3] However, elderly persons with low dietary diversity scores have a high risk that their basic skills will decrease rapidly as they age (Kumagai 2011) (Fig. 4.1). In addition, their poor nutritional condition will decrease serum albumin in elderly persons. Serum albumin is necessary for the maintenance of good health. The investigation of food diversity was performed by Japanese nutritionists using long-standing panel surveys; therefore, this investigatory survey is useful for measuring elderly persons' healthy eating behaviors.

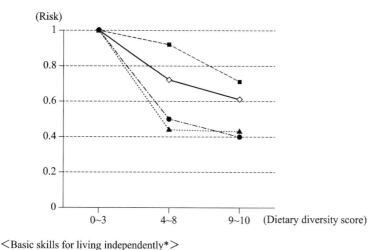

<Basic skills for living independently*>

—◇— Total score   --■-- Instrumental activities for daily living
--●-- Intellectual activities   ····▲···· Social role

* The Tokyo metropolitan institute gerontology index of competence in community-dwelling older people independent in daily living

Fig. 4.1 Relationship between old person's risk to decrease basic skills for living independently and dietary diversity score. *Source* Kumagai et al. (2003)

4.2   Distribution of Urban Food Deserts in Tokyo and Minato Ward's Characteristics

As we mentioned in Chap. 3, Sect. 3.1, it is possible to make food access maps using a geographical information system (GIS). A wide range of food access maps from micro scale (city and town scale maps) to macro scale (e.g., Tokyo Metropolitan Area scale maps) are available.

Figure 4.2 is a food access map of the 23 special Tokyo wards. This map is based on the 2005 Japanese national census. Some geographical methods are available for measuring food accessibility. In this chapter, we calculated poor food access areas by comparing the balance between the demand for foods (the number of elderly persons over 65 years old) and supply of foods (the number of food retailers, such as supermarkets and grocers). In particular, we measured the residents' accessibility to

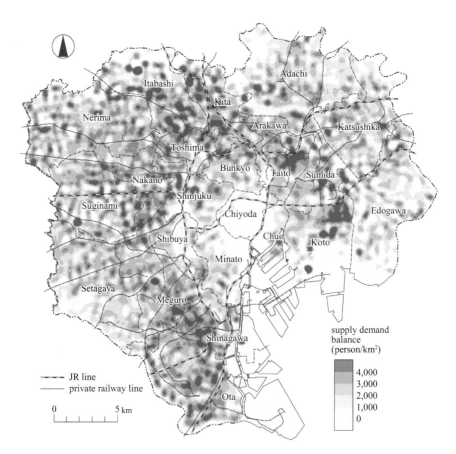

Fig. 4.2 Distribution of shopping disadvantaged old people in Tokyo 23 wards in 2005. *Source* Iwama et al. (2011)

food retailers using kernel density estimation to quantitatively define the urban food deserts. We previously explained the kernel density estimation in detail in Chap. 3, Sect. 3.1.

In Fig. 4.2, areas with high positive values indicate areas of excessive demand. There are many disadvantaged consumers in the excessive demand areas; e.g., many disadvantaged consumers are shown in the wards of Koto, Taito, Arakawa, Itabashi, Nakano, and Meguro. However, shopping environments are easily changed by local traffic conditions, residents' characteristics (e.g., age, social class, car ownership, income), administrative support, food retailers' delivery services, and so on. Field surveys are necessary to correctly understand the study area's shopping environments. Minato Ward is mainly a business district with relatively few residents; however, there may be an insufficient number of food retailers in some areas of this ward.

Figure 4.3 shows the urban food deserts in Minato Ward; e.g., some areas including District A are urban food deserts, while there are statistically few shopping-disadvantaged people in District B.

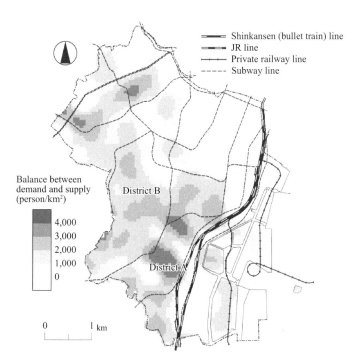

Fig. 4.3 Distribution of shopping disadvantaged old people in Minato ward in 2005. *Source* Iwama et al. (2011)

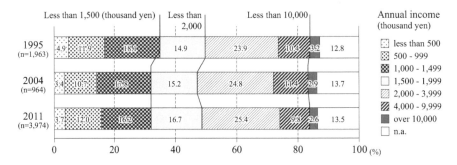

Fig. 4.4 Average annual income of old single households in Minato ward. *Source* Kawai (2015)

4.3   Residents and Elderly Persons' Poverty

As mentioned in Chapter 2, many elderly persons live in central Tokyo (see Fig. 2.8) in addition to a diverse variety of people. Thus, the population composition of central Tokyo continues to diversify. Single elderly people living alone in central Tokyo have many kinds of neighbors, such as young people aged in their 20s, white-collar single women with a high educational background, and foreigners (see Figs. 2.11–2.16). The same tendency can be observed in Minato Ward. In those areas where diverse types of people live together, the residents' lifestyles and values are very different; therefore, it is very difficult for those areas' local communities to create social capital. In short, local communities tend to be weaker in central Tokyo, including Minato Ward, than other areas and elderly urban residents have a high risk of being isolated from their local communities.

Although Minato Ward is one of the richest areas of central Tokyo, the number of elderly persons in poverty living in this ward is increasing. In the 2015 national census, Minato Ward residents' average income was 10.2 million yen, while the national average income is about 4.1 million yen. Thus, many high-income residents clearly live in Minato Ward. However, Kawai (2015) studied elderly persons' living environment in Minato Ward and found that almost half had suffered from poverty. He also clarified that about 30% of single elderly persons were living at a minimum standard of living (e.g., less than 1.5 million yen per year) (Fig. 4.4).

4.4   District A Case Study

4.4.1   Method

In this section, we analyze the relationship between elderly persons' eating habits and residents' attributes using a questionnaire survey. The District A study area appears to include many disadvantaged shoppers. We performed a questionnaire survey in 2010 with the research object being all households who live in some postcode areas of the post office branch A (a total of 21,430 households).[4] In total, 2,660 households responded, with a 12.4% collection rate. There were 2,527 valid responses and 883 were from elderly persons over 65 years old. The main purpose of this book is to discuss the food desert issues of elderly persons in Japan. Therefore, in subsection 3, "research results," we analyze the residents' attributes of all households (2,527 families). And in subsection 4, "the relationship between the elderly persons' eating habits and personal attributes," we analyzed just 883 samples (i.e., the sample of persons aged over 6 5 years old).

4.4.2 District A Outline

An outline of District A i s shown in Fig. 4.5. District A (a-*cho*,[5] b-*cho*, c-*cho*, d-*cho*, e-*cho*, and f-*cho*) is located around a JR (Japan Railway) station. District A is divided into higher ground on the Musashino Plateau (a, b) and lower ground on the seaside (b–f).

During early modern times, many feudal lords had their suburban residences in this area, and these areas are now used by upmarket residential districts, hotels, big box retailers, and universities (Photo 4.1). The lower ground faces Tokyo Bay and

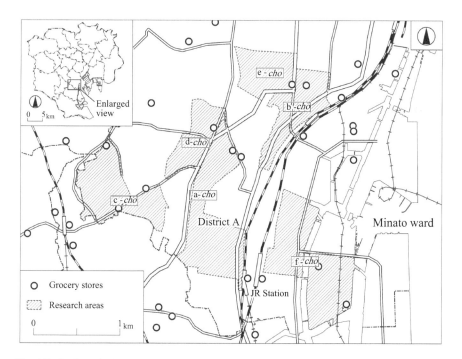

Fig. 4.5 Outline of District A in 2010. *Source* Asakawa (2013)

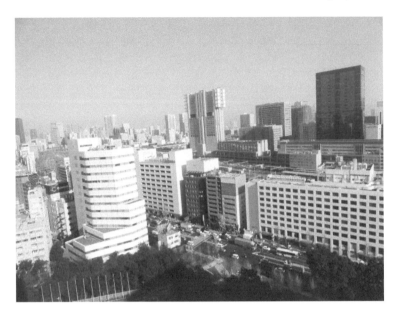

Photo 4.1 Big box retailers in front of A station (District A, 2011, taken by Iwama)

was formerly a landfill site. Many seaside distribution warehouses used to be in this area. This seaside area recently became very popular and many apartment towers have been built (Photos 4.2 and 4.3). However, many old-fashioned houses, elderly shopping streets, and factories can still be found in District A, d-*cho* (Photos 4.4 and 4.5).

4.4.3   Questionnaire Survey Results (Simple Totaling)

First, we produced outlines of elderly persons aged over 65 years old by analyzing their living environment using the questionnaire survey results. Table 4.1 shows the personal attributes of questionnaire respondents. More than 60% of the respondents were women. Although many of the respondents were aged in their 30s and 60s, we obtained questionnaire responses from a wide range of age groups. Considering the family structure, the proportion of single households was the highest (34.7%). Elderly persons living with their children (31.5%) and couple households (29.1%) were the next highest after single households. Considering education background, the proportion of university graduates was the highest (44.0%). Considering household income, 20% stated that they earned "from 3 to 4.99 million yen per year," while 23% indicated "less than 2 million yen per year." Many elderly persons who live only on their pension were in this category. On the one hand, some families' incomes appear to be low, but they have many assets tied up in properties and deeds. On the other

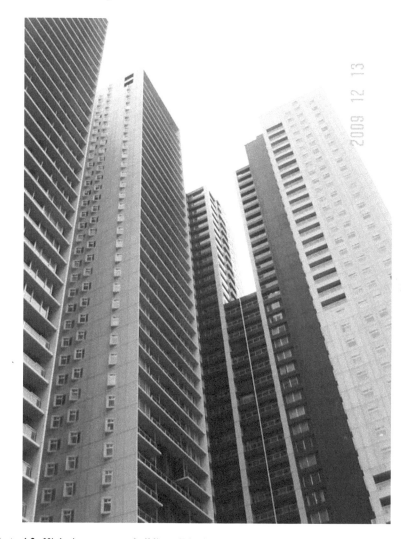

Photo 4.2 High-rise apartment buildings (District A-f, 2009, taken by Iwama)

hand, the proportion of high-income families with 10 million yen was also high (27%).

Next, we outlined the living environments using the questionnaire results (Table 4.2). Considering living place, we received many questionnaires from respondents in a-*cho*. Considering the house ownership, the largest percentage of answers comprised "self-possession: multiple-dwelling type" and "self-possession: single house" with high scores (14.0%). However, the proportion of respondents who indicated "rental: apartment house built by the Japanese Housing Corp" and "rental: apartment house built by the government," whose rents are lower, were also relatively high in both categories (in total, 19.0%). Considering years of residence, 40.6% of

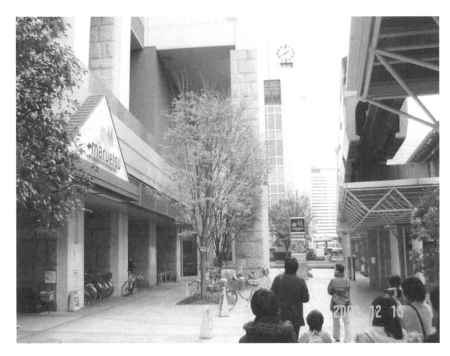

Photo 4.3 Grocery store adjacent to High-rise apartment buildings (District A-f, 2009, taken by Iwama)

respondents were categorized as "less than 5 years." However, those who indicated "more than 20 years" also showed a high score (27.5%). Considering the respondents' previous address, many answered with "Minato Ward" or "23 Tokyo wards." Many respondents intended to live in urban areas. Minato Ward is especially popular and 90% of the respondents hoped to keep living in Minato Ward. Considering shopping behaviors, 29% responded "almost every day," 37% indicated "3–5 times per week," 30% "1–2 times per week" and 4% "1–3 times per month."

We then analyzed elderly persons' eating habits to measure their malnutrition risk. This investigation focused on elderly persons aged over 65 years; therefore, we narrowed down our survey target to respondents aged over 65 years and investigated their food diversity. As a result, about 44.6% of elderly persons fell under the limit (less than a score of 4) (Table 4.3). In general, men's scores were worse than women's scores. In the case of men, the percentage who had limited food diversity was 53.6%.

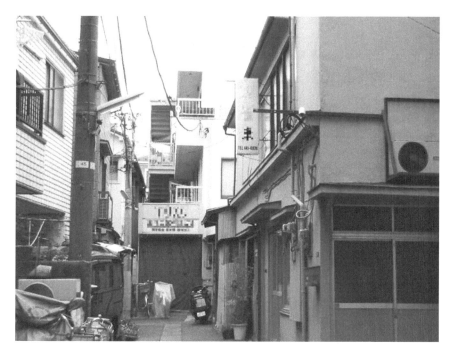

Photo 4.4 Old-fashioned houses and factories (District A-d, 2009, taken by Asakawa)

4.4.4   The Relationship Between Elderly Persons' Eating Habits and Group Participation (E.g., Club Activities, Neighborhood Associations)

To clarify the relationship between elderly persons' eating habits and social capital at the regional level, we analyzed the respondents' public participation. Club activities, such as sports, hobbies, cultural school, and social activities, such as neighborhood associations, were important opportunities for elderly persons to keep in touch with their local communities. In our questionnaire, we asked each elderly person some questions about their participation in these groups. As a result, 29.1% of respondents had not participated in any groups, while 28.4% joined just one group, and 42.4% had participated in more than two groups.

We analyzed the relationship between elderly persons' eating habits and group participation. As a result, we found a statistically significant relationship in women: i.e., 47.8% of women who participated in no group were classified with a high risk of malnutrition (less than a score of 4). Only 32.7% of women who participated in one or more groups were classified with a high risk of malnutrition. In the case of men, however, we could not find any statistically significant relationship between their eating habits and group participation. Thus, women's eating habits are strongly defined by their public participation.

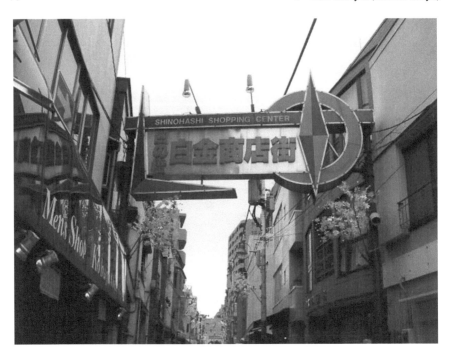

Photo 4.5   Older hopping streets (District A-d, 2009, taken by Asakawa)

4.4.5   The Relationship Between Eating Habits and Social Networks

Next, to identify respondents' social networks (e.g., their ties with family, friends, and colleagues), we investigated the number of closest people and their social attributes. The question, "can you unburden your troubles and discontentment to them?" is an important index for judging whether the respondent has close relations with their "closest people" or not. First, we asked the respondents about the number of people to whom they can unburden their troubles and discontentment, including their partners. As a result, 49.3% of respondents answered "0–3 people." Therefore, if we asked each respondent to list up to three of their closest people, we can obtain almost half of their social network.

Therefore, we asked each respondent to list up to three of their closest people, including their partner, and about their relationship with them. In particular, we classified these three closest people into seven categories: "a person who lives in a distant place," "a friend from school," "family and relatives," "a member of the same club," "a neighbor," "a former work buddy," and "a specialist, such as doctor, care worker, or nursery teacher." As a result, 75.3% of elderly persons listed more than one of "a member of the same club" as their closest friends, while 66.7% responded "a friend from school" and 53.3% responded "family and relatives." "A specialist"

Table 4.1 Personal attributes of questionnaire respondents

Gender		Age		Family type		Academic background		Household income	
Male	37.1	20–29	5.0	Single	34.7	High school	22.0	Less than 1.0 (million yen)	5.0
Female	62.9	30–39	19.0	Couple	29.1	Technical school	8.0	1.0–2.9	18.0
		40–49	17.0	With one's own parents	4.7	Junior college	12.0	3.0–4.9	20.0
		50–59	14.0	With one's own children	31.5	Technical college	2.0	5.0–6.9	14.0
		60–69	20.0			University	44.0	7.0–9.9	16.0
		70–79	17.0			Graduate school	7.0	10.0–14.9	14.0
		Over 80 years old	8.0			Others	5.0	15.0–19.9	7.0
								20.0–29.9	4.0
								Over 30.0	2.0

Source Ishii (2013)

Table 4.2 Living environments of questionnaire respondents

(%)

Living place		House ownership		Years of residence		Previous address		Preferred residential area	
a-cho	26.0	Self-possession: single house	14.0	Less than 2 year	23.7	Current address	7.1	Strongly desire to live in current address	46.1
b-cho	9.3	Self-possession: multiple-dwelling house	43.0	3–5 year	16.9	Minato Ward	21.6	Want to live in current address	44.1
c-cho	12.3	Rental: apartment house	21.0	6–9 year	12.7	23 Tokyo Wards	44.2	Want to move to other place	8.0
d-cho	16.5	Rental: apartment house built by the Japanese Housing Crop	3.0	10–19 year	17.3	Tokyo metropolitan area	3.2	Strongly desire to move to other place	1.8
e-cho	12.9	Rental: apartment house built by the government	16.0	20–49 year	21.1	Other areas in Japan	21.7		
f-cho	23.0	Company housing	4.0	over 50 year	6.4	Oversea	2.2		
		Other	1.0						

Source Ishii (2013)

Table 4.3 Food diversity scores (by gender and age)

	Age composition	Elderly people with diversity scores over 4 (%)	Elderly people with diversity scores less than 4 (%)
Male	60–69	46.7	53.3
	70–79	43.9	56.1
	Over 80 years old	51.4	48.6
	Total	46.4	53.6
Female	60–69	50.0	50.0
	70–79	63.8	36.2
	Over 80 years old	67.2	32.8
	Total	60.9	39.1
Total		55.4	44.6

$n = 881$
Source Ishii (2013)

Table 4.4 Result of principal component analysis

	The primary component	The second component	The third component
A person who lives in a distant place	0.59	−0.32	0.09
A friend from school	0.58	−0.44	−0.02
Family and relatives	0.52	0.33	0.36
A member of the same club	0.49	−0.28	−0.38
A neighbor	0.48	0.45	−0.27
A former work buddy	0.26	0.55	−0.40
A specialist	0.26	0.19	0.71
Characteristic value	1.56	1.03	1.02
Contribution ratio (%)	22.34	14.65	14.59
Cumulative contribution ratio (%)	22.34	36.99	51.58

Source Asakawa (2013)

was listed by 7.2% of elderly persons. These results suggest that in general, the elderly persons' closest friend was "a member of the same club" and followed by "a friend from school" and "family and relatives."

We performed a principal component analysis to organize these close relationships (Table 4.4). As a result, the primary component shows high loads in the seven categories. Therefore, we named the primary component "various networks." The second component shows positive high loads for "a neighbor" and "a former work buddy," and it also showed negative high loads for "a person who lives in a distant place" and "a friend from school." Therefore, we named the second component "the network focusing on workplace." The third component showed negative high loads for "a member of the same club" and "a former work buddy," and it also showed positive high loads for "a specialist." Therefore, we named the third component, "specialist network." In short, the primary component showed the respondents' networks with their families, neighbors, and friends. The second component was the interaction with a former work buddy, while the third component is the interaction with specialists, such as doctors and care workers.

We calculated the principal component scores. Then, using a *t*-test, we checked the differences between the average scores of respondents with high or low malnutrition risk. As a result, we found statistically significant differences in the primary component. That is, the respondents who do not have a wide range of interactions are at high risk for deteriorating healthy eating habits.

4.4.6   Unfavorable Factors for Elderly Persons' Eating Habits

What kind of elderly persons tend to have deteriorated healthy eating habits? To answer this question from a wide perspective, we performed a logistic regression separated by men and women. The research indicators are personal attributes (e.g., age, family component, living place, income), group participation (e.g., the number of neighborhood association activities and club activities they participate in), and social networks (i.e., the principal component scores). The results for women are shown in Table 4.5 and in the following:

1.   As people get a year old, the risk of malnutrition will decrease 7%.
2.   Compared with middle-class people, low-income (less than 3 million yen per year) people's malnutrition risk is 1.8 times higher, while high-income (more than 10 million yen per year) people's malnutrition risk is 2.1 times higher.
3.   The malnutrition risk for people who do not participate in any group activities are 1.9 times higher than those of people who participate in some activities.
4.   People with various networks tend to have a low risk of malnutrition.

It is difficult to understand why high-income people are at high risk of malnutrition. However, wealthy people tend to pay excessive attention to healthy eating with extreme diet and dietary restrictions. We should investigate this question carefully through interview surveys to prove this tentative theory.

Next, the results for men are shown in Table 4.6. We found the following tendencies:

1.   As people age, the risk of malnutrition will decrease 4%.
2.   The malnutrition risks for respondents with families are 55% lower than those of single people.

Table 4.5 Result of logistic regression analysis (female)

	Coefficient of regression	Odds ratio
Age	−0.07	0.93**
Living place		
a-*cho*	0.12	1.13
b-*cho*	0.15	1.16
c-*cho*	−0.40	0.67
d-*cho*	−0.07	0.94
e-*cho*	0.15	1.17
Family income		
Less than 3.0 (million yen)	0.59	1.80*
More than 10.0 (million yen)	0.76	2.13*
Number of activities		
0	0.61	1.85*
1	0.44	1.56
Live with one's own children	−0.24	0.78
Single household	−0.24	0.79
The principal component scores	−0.25	0.78*
Constants	4.19	66.02

Note Basic categories are as follow:
Living place: Konan1, 4-*chome*
Family income: 3.0–10.0 million yen
The number of activities: more than one
Live with one's own children: yes
Single household: yes
Model $\chi 2$ score $= 41.9\ df = 13\ p < .01$
R^2 score $= .113$
**$p < .01$ *$p < .05$
Source Asakawa (2013)

4.4.7 Living Environment for Elderly Persons in District A

The above results show that nearly 44.6% of elderly persons clearly have bad eating habits and face a high risk of malnutrition. Compared with women, men clearly have a higher risk of malnutrition. The factors that mainly cause worse eating habits differ by sex. For women, participating in groups and maintaining various social networks were important in preventing malnutrition. However, for men, the existence of their family living together was very important for maintaining their good eating habits. Nevertheless, not only poor people whose annual incomes were less than 3 million yen, but also high-income earners whose annual incomes were over 10 million yen also tend to have unbalanced diets and risk malnutrition. We can easily understand

Table 4.6 Result of logistic regression analysis (male)

	Coefficient of regression	Odds ratio
Age	−0.04	0.96*
Family income		
Less than 3.0 (million yen)	0.08	1.08
More than 10.0 (million yen)	−0.01	0.99
Live with one's own children	−0.23	0.80
Single household	−0.79	0.45*
The principal component scores	−0.15	0.86
Constants	3.77	43.17

Note Basic categories are as follow:
Family income: 3.0–10.0 million yen
Live with one's own children: yes
Single household: yes
Model $\chi 2$ score $= 41.9$ $df = 13$ $p < .01$
R^2 score $= .113$
$**p < .01; *p < .05$
Source Asakawa (2013)

the relationship between poverty and poor diet, but the cause-and-effect relationship between high-income earners and poor diet is unclear. Further investigation is necessary to answer this question.

4.5   District B Case Study

4.5.1   Method

In this section, we analyze the relationship between elderly persons' eating habits and resident attributes in District B. Shoppers in this district appear to be less disadvantaged than shoppers in District A. We performed a questionnaire survey from April 2 to 14, 2012. District B is a business area with many public institutions, embassies, and offices. We chose some residential areas in District B: g-*cho* (832 families, 1,571 people, with a rate of aging at around 19.3%); h-*cho* (947 families, 1,348 people, rate of aging around 17.6%); and i-*cho* (1,012 families, 1,176 people, rate of aging around 6.8%). The questionnaire was delivered to all households in the postal delivery area. In addition, the post office also delivered the remaining questionnaires to other areas within District B. The questionnaire comprised nine questions about personal attributes (e.g., family structure, education background, household income), four questions about living place (e.g., dwelling history, reason for selection, whether they wanted to stay there longer or not, and regional problems), nine questions about shopping behaviors (e.g., means of accessing stores, shopping frequency, transit time, do they use food delivery services or not), one question about eating habits (food diversity), two questions about health (instrumental activities of daily living[6]), and two questions about local community ties (e.g., group participation, interactions with neighbors[7]). These questions are widely used in sociology and nutrition science. The validity of these questions has been proved by these disciplines. In addition, Fig. 4.3 shows that District B's shopping environment is sufficient; therefore, we did not investigate food access in this district.

District B residents are relatively young; therefore, the valid response was 201 out of 3,867 households with a collection rate of 5.2% (although the collection rate from elderly persons was 10.5%). In general, obtaining answers from working people who live in urban areas is difficult and we could not collect sufficient responses from District B respondents. Thus, our research results might not show the collective characteristics of this district. However, we can understand the outline of District B using this questionnaire survey.

Because the collection rate for this questionnaire survey was not sufficient, it is impossible to use statistical methods such as multilevel surveys and multiple regression analysis. In this section, we therefore investigated the residents' personal attributes, shopping environments, living environments, group participation, and interaction with their neighbors using a simple tabulation and logistic regression. Based on these results, we discussed the relationship between elderly persons' eating habits and their personal and social attributes.

4.5.2 District B Outline

Figure 4.6 shows the outline for District B (g, h, i, j, k, and l-*cho*). This district is in an undulating area with hills and valleys called Yamanote. The population of this district is 466,602 with a 16.1% rate of aging (2005 national census). In the Edo era, many *daimyō*'s suburban residences, temples, and shrines were built on the hill-top plateaus while craftsman lived in residential districts in the valleys. These sites are now upmarket residential districts with embassies (Photo 4.6). This district recently became a special residential area for famous celebrities with many upmarket shopping streets and supermarkets (Photo 4.7). Thus, food access is sufficient in this district. However, because these stores provide luxury foods, these shopping environments may not be convenient for middle- and low-income households.

District B is very popular for emerging celebrities; however, it is very difficult for elderly residents with an average income to keep living in this area because of the soaring land prices and expensive fixed property and inheritance taxes. Therefore, many elderly residents had already moved out of the area by the 1980s. Some elderly residents kept their residence only in areas h and j.

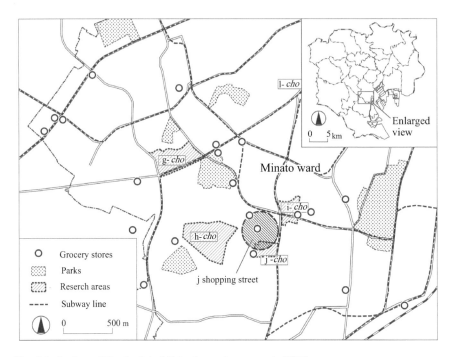

Fig. 4.6 Outline of District B in 2011. *Source* Iwama et al. (2011)

4.5.3   Questionnaire Survey Results (Simple Totaling)

Table 4.7 shows the results of our food diversity investigation using our questionnaire survey. Around 55.2% of the elderly persons fell under the limit (less than a score of 4). It is surprising that many elderly residents suffer from malnutrition risk in this rich and food-convenient area. Moreover, the malnutrition risk in District B was higher than that in District A, although the food access in District B is higher than in District A. Some respondents commented that the nearby stores were too expensive for them to buy food daily. In central Tokyo, we must consider not only physical access to grocery stores, but also the price range for foods.

Table 4.8 shows the respondents' personal attributes: e.g., 72.4% of the respondents were women. Although many of the respondents were aged in their 40s and 70s, we obtained responses to the questionnaire from a wide range of age groups. Considering the family structure, the proportions of single households, couple households, and families with their children were over 30% respectively. Many single households are elderly persons who lost their partner. Many families have young children who are not yet independent from their parents. Considering the respondents' education background, some elderly residents were high school graduates, but almost all of the younger generation have higher education, such as university undergraduates or master's and doctoral graduates. Considering income, clear bipolarization could be

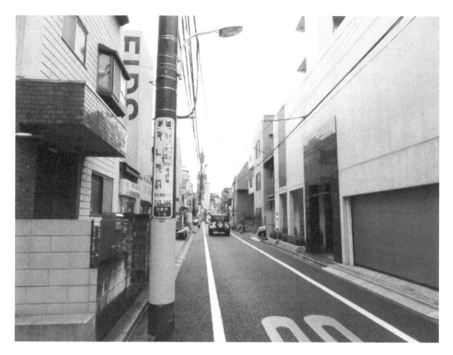

Photo 4.6 Upmarket residential districts (District B, 2011, taken by Iwama)

observed: e.g., the number of families whose annual income is from 3 to 4.99 million yen was 37.5%.[8] However, the proportion of high-income families with an income over 10 million yen is also high (36.3%).

Next, Table 4.9 outlines the respondents' living environments. Questionnaires were almost uniformly received from all areas (g–j). The post officers randomly delivered the remaining questionnaires in areas k and l; therefore, the number of responses from these areas were relatively small.

Considering home ownership, the largest percentage of answers was "self-possession (single house and multiple-dwelling type)" at 59.7%. However, "rental: apartment house built by the Japanese Housing Corp" and "rental: apartment house built by the government" were also relatively high (40.3% in total). Considering years of residence, 32.8% of respondents were categorized as "less than 5 years," while "more than 30 years" also showed a high score (26.9%). Considering the respondents' former address, 6.6% answered "born and grown up in the same place." Most responses were from "Minato Ward" (24.9%) or "23 Tokyo wards" (40.5%). Some residents were foreigners, with 2.5% indicating "overseas." District B is not only a convenient area, but also a high-status residential area; therefore, 90% of residents hope to keep living in this district.

Table 4.10 shows the respondents' shopping behaviors. The survey items about shopping behaviors were a little bit different between questionnaire surveys in Districts A and B. 11.2 and 64.8% consider their shopping environment as being

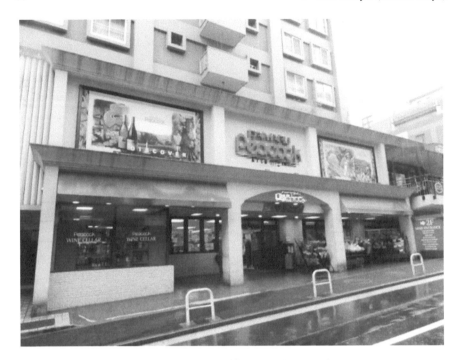

Photo 4.7 Upmarket supermarkets (District B, 2011, taken by Iwama)

Table 4.7 Food diversity scores

Low score group (less than 3.0)	55.2%
High score group (4.0 or higher)	44.8%
Average score	3.9

Source Iwama et al. (2011)

"uncomfortable" or "comfortable," respectively. The shopping frequency is relatively high and many respondents went shopping on foot. In general, the physical shopping environment (food access) of District B appears not to be poor. Nevertheless, some respondents answered that they are not rich enough to purchase food daily at their neighboring luxury grocery shops.

Table 4.11 shows the respondents' participation in clubs, such as sports, cultural schools, parent–teacher associations (e.g., class mother), and neighborhood associations. Many working households live in this district; therefore, only 31.5% answered "no group participation." However, 23.4 and 21.3% of respondents participated in one or two groups, respectively. These groups were mainly sports clubs and cultural schools. This suggests that District B residents do not participate in local activities. Nevertheless, although the number is small, a few residents joined many local activities. Some of them were the president of an art club, directors of incorporated nonprofit organizations, a senior church member, or director of a sports association.

Table 4.8 Personal attributes of questionnaire respondents

Gender		Age		Family type		Academic background		Household income	
Male	27.6	Less than 10	1.5	Single	30.5	High school	19.5	Less than 1.0 (million yen)	3.8
Female	72.4	20–29	5.5	Couple	30.5	Technical school	6.0	1.0–2.9	12.5
		30–39	13.4	With one's own children	31.5	Junior college	10.5	3.0–4.9	19.4
		40–49	20.4	Other	7.5	Technical college	1.5	5.0–6.9	12.5
		50–59	14.9			University	43.0	7.0–9.9	13.8
		60–69	19.4			Graduate school	4.0	10.0–14.9	16.9
		70–79	21.4					15.0–19.9	7.5
		Over 80 years old	3.5					20.0–29.9	5.6
								Over 30.0	6.3

Note figures are %
Source Iwama et al. (2011)

Table 4.9 Living environments of questionnaire respondents

Living place		House ownership		Years of residence		Previous address		Hope of future habitation	
g-cho	22.4	Self-possession: Single house	28.9	Less than 5 year	32.8	Current address	6.6	Strongly desire to live in current address	48.4
h-cho	22.4	Self-possession: Multiple-dwelling house	19.9	6–10 year	10.9	Minato Ward	24.9		
i-cho	28.9	Rental: apartment House	32.8	11–15 year	14.8	23 Tokyo Wards	40.5	Want to live in current address	42.1
j-cho	19.9	Rental: apartment house built by the Japanese Housing Crop	2.0	16–20 year	4.9	Tokyo Pref.	3.5		
k-cho	3.0	Rental: apartment house built by the government	0.5	21–25 year	3.8	Other areas in Japan	22.0	Want to move to other place	7.9
l-cho	2.5	Company housing	2.5	26–30 year	6.0	Oversea	2.5		
No data	1.0	Other	2.5	31–35 year	2.2			Strongly desire to move to other place	1.6
				36–40 year	5.5				
				41–45 year	6.6				
				46–50 year	4.4				
				Over 50 year	8.2				

Source Iwama et al. (2011)

Table 4.10 Shopping behavior

Shopping environment		Frequency of self-cooking		Shopping frequency		Main transportation to go shopping	
Inconvenient	11.2	Everyday	69.7	Everyday	18.9	On foot	61.3
Somewhat inconvenient	24.0	3–5 times per week	16.9	3–5 times per week	37.3	By bicycle	12.1
Somewhat convenient	33.2	1–2 times per week	8.0	1–2 times per week	36.8	By bus	2.0
Convenient	31.6	1–3 times per month	1.5	1–3 times per month	4.0	By taxi	1.5
		Others	4.0	Others	3.0	By train	1.5
						By car/motorcycle (drive by myself)	6.5
						By car/motorcycle (drive by family members)	3.0
						Home delivery	2.0
						Other	10.1

Note Figures are %
Source Iwama et al. (2011)

Table 4.11 Number of respondents' participation in clubs

(%)			
Score		Score	
0	31.5	6	1.5
1	23.4	7	0.5
2	21.3	8	0.0
3	9.1	9	1.5
4	6.6	10	0.5
5	4.1		

Source Iwama et al. (2011)

These people are usually elderly residents and their relationships with their local community are in complete contrast to those of new residents.

Table 4.12 shows respondents' interactions with their neighbors. Many residents are isolated from their local communities; e.g., 82.8% answered that they "say hello to their neighbors." Only 61.6% "know their neighbor's family construction" and 49.7% "know their neighbor household's occupation." In addition, merely 29.1% of residents "gave souvenirs to neighbors or get souvenirs from their neighbors," 19.2%

Table 4.12 Respondents' interactions with their neighbors (the ratio of their answer 'yes')

(%)		
(1)	Say hello to their neighbors	82.9
(2)	Visit their neighbors houses or invite neighbors to their house	21.7
(3)	Know their neighbor's family construction	61.6
(4)	Know their neighbor householder's occupation	49.7
(5)	Gave souvenirs to neighbors or get souvenirs from their neighbors	29.1
(6)	Talk to their neighbors about their concerns	19.2
(7)	Borrow something (i.e. seasonings such as soy source) from their neighbors or lend something to neighbors	11.1
(8)	Go out with their neighbors	10.6
(9)	Go on a journey with their neighbors	5.6
(10)	Relatives	2.6
(11)	No one live	5.1

Source Iwama et al. (2011)

"talk to their neighbors about their concerns," and 10.6% "go out with their neighbors." These scores are much lower than for other places where we have researched previously.[9]

4.5.4   Elderly Persons' Unhealthy Eating Habits

To investigate elderly persons' unhealthy eating habits, we performed a logistic regression survey. The explained variable was "the food diversity score" and the explanatory variables were "age," "sex," "family structure," "shopping environment" (whether they feel uncomfortable, or not), "group participation" (the number of neighborhood association and club activities they participate in), and "their tie with neighbors" (whether the questionnaires know the next-door neighbor's family construction or not) (Table 4.13). Because of high missing values, we deleted "family income" from the explanatory variables. As a result, we found a statistically significant relationship only with "age" and "sex."

1. Elderly persons have a higher risk of malnutrition than younger people.
2. Men have a higher risk of malnutrition than women.

   The number of samples is relatively small in District B. In this case study, the explanatory variables related to social capital ("group participation" and "ties with neighbors") did not have a statistically significant correlation with the "food diversity score." However, the odds ratio suggests that social capital has some influence on elderly persons' healthy eating habits. In addition, interview surveys from residents showed that newcomers who created their wealth in one generation and moved to this district tend to be richer than the former residents. Newcomers generally have

Table 4.13 Result of logistic regression analysis (the reasons of old people's bad eating habits)

	Coefficient of regression	Odds ratio
Age	−0.173	0.841*
Gender	2.047	7.743*
Family structure		
Couple household	−0.307	0.735
With their children	−1.547	0.213
Others	−0.157	0.854
Shopping environment		
In convenient	0.484	1.622
Somewhat inconvenient	1.193	3.296
Convenient	−0.011	0.989
The number of activities		
0	0.429	1.536
1	−0.83	0.436
Interactions with their neighbors	1.105	3.02
Constants	12.365	*

Note Basic categories are as follow:
Gender: female
Family structure: single household
Shopping environment: convenient
The number of activities: more than one
Interactions with their neighbors: 'I know their neighbor's family construction'
Model $\chi 2$ score $= 20.1$ $df = 11$ $p < .05$
R^2 score $= .277$
*$p < .05$
Source Iwama et al. (2011)

weak ties to their local communities. Although we could not show clear evidence, "income" might be also an important explanatory variable in District B (because "income" is a significant explanatory variable in the District A case study).

4.5.5 Living Environment in District B

The knowledge that we obtained from this case study follows. First, District B has a good shopping environment. However, around 55.6% of elderly residents suffer from a high malnutrition risk because of their unhealthy eating habits. Although the shopping environment in District B was better than that of District A, the malnutrition risk in District B was higher than that in District A. We investigated the relationship between elderly persons' eating habits and their personal attributes. As a result, we found that elderly persons' sex and ages have a statistically significant relationship with their eating habits. Moreover, group participation and communication among neighbors also have a strong influence on healthy eating habits.

However, we could not gain a high-enough response rate; therefore, these results may not have geographical representativeness. We should perform an additional investigation to correctly understand the characteristics of urban food deserts in central Tokyo.

4.6   Summary

In this chapter, we discussed the characteristics of urban food deserts in the case study areas of Districts A and B in Minato Ward, Tokyo. Both districts include many upmarket residential areas, but although many luxury grocers exist in these districts, we found little availability of food access areas in the business districts near major railway stations and the reclaimed land at the seaside.

Minato Ward is generally considered as a celebrity area free from social exclusion, such as food deserts. However, we found that many elderly residents suffer from high malnutrition risk (District A: 44.6%; District B: 55.2%). This study clarified that personal attributes, such as sex (women) and age, have a statistically significant relationship with healthy eating habits. In addition, the ties with families and neighbors (group participation and communication among neighbors), and family income (less than 3 million yen and over 10 million yen per year) also have a strong influence on healthy eating. Thus, not only personal attributes, but also social capital and income control elderly persons' healthy eating habits. This knowledge also means that the respondents' isolation from their families and local communities may possibly cause malnutrition in elderly residents and create urban food deserts.

Urban city centers, such as central Tokyo, are at serious risk of urban food desert issues expanding widely among isolated elderly persons. However, few studies have explored urban food deserts and its characteristics are not clear. We must investigate this issue from interdisciplinary perspectives to clarify the actual condition of urban food deserts in Japan.

Notes

1. According to interview surveys, the incomes of elderly residents are not high. However, many have inherited real estate and receive unearned income from these properties. Nevertheless, it may become difficult for elderly residents on standard incomes to pay the fixed property taxes on their properties that are increasing in value. Therefore, these respondents sold their land and moved to other areas.
2. Almost half of elderly residents are living in poverty. Many of them lived in Minato Ward before the so-called "bubble" economic era in the 1980s when land prices in this area rapidly increased and Minato Ward became a luxury residential area. In general, elderly persons and low-income families tend to

stay in the same place for a long time. While many high-rise condominiums for rich residents were built together in large numbers, low-rise wooden houses for low-income elderly residents still exist in the same area. On the one hand, the average price of seaside high-rise condominiums is more than one hundred million yen. On the other hand, the average house rent for old public housings are about thirty thousand yen per month. Thus, bipolarization can be seen in the residents of this ward and is especially clear among elderly residents.

3. 'Instrumental activities for daily living' are fundamental for elderly people to remain independent in daily life. If elderly people have reduced ability to perform instrumental activities, it will become difficult for them to do domestic tasks such as cooking and cleaning, or to manage finances. 'Intellectual activities' require the ability to search for, create, or participate in leisure activities. Intellectual activities require sophisticated thought. This ability is the core of people's attractiveness and dignity. If elderly people's intellectual abilities are reduced, they tend to pass time in useless ways, without purpose. 'Social role' requires the ability to cherish other people. This ability has a strong relationship with elderly people's consideration for others, kindness in giving advice and guidance, and positive interactions with young people. If the ability to fulfil this role is reduced, it becomes difficult for them to maintain relationships with neighbors or to perform important social activities such as participating in neighborhood associations.

4. We chose the research areas randomly from all postcode areas of the post office branch A and the study period was from November 15 to December 25, 2010.

5. Japanese address system is different from those of European countries. Although European address systems are usually based on street, Japanese system is mainly based on town block "cho".

6. This index measures elderly persons' ability necessary for living in society. This index was developed by Tokyo Metropolitan Geriatric Hospital. This index is similar to "activities of daily living"; it can measure not only basic activity of daily living, but also high-level abilities such as means of self-reliance, knowledge initiatives, and social roles.

7. This is a kind of index that measures the local level of social capital. Please see Chap. 3, Sect. 3.2 for more details.

8. Many low-income households are elderly people with pensions as their main income. In general, however, elderly persons have sufficient savings and own property. These elderly persons appear not to suffer extreme poverty.

9. Knowing their neighbor's family construction is a very important index for judging their ties with their neighbors. Our previous studies clarified that even if elderly persons do not have an intimate relationship with their neighbors, they are not totally isolated from their community if moderate ties are kept with their neighbors, such as "know their neighbor's family construction." These elderly persons' risk of malnutrition is not as high.

References

Asakawa T (2013) The phase of social relationships and food deserts problem: the comparison between MINATO Ward, Tokyo and Sata, Kagoshima Prefecture. Bull Inst Sociol Soc Work, Meiji Gakuin Univ 43:147–156 (Japanese)

Ishii D (2013) The survey report of the residents in Minato Ward: analyses of relationships with important others and everyday's meals. Bull Inst Sociol Soc Work, Meiji Gakuin Univ 43:91–108 (Japanese)

Iwama N, Tanaka K, Sasaki M, Komaki N (2011) The isolation of the elderly households and the deterioration of their life environment in the urban renewal area of central Tokyo. Japan Geographic Data Center Academic Research Grant Report in 2011 (Japanese). http://www.kokudo.or.jp/grant/pdf/h23/iwama.pdf. Accessed 14 Aug 2020

Kawai K (2015) Japan: the country which is not nice to old people. Kobunsha Co., Ltd, Tokyo (Japanese)

Kumagai S (2011) Stop eating poor meal for the prevention of nursing care (Kaigo Saretakunai nara Soshoku ha yamenasai). Kodansha LTD, Tokyo

Kumagai S, Watanabe S, Shibata H, Amano H, Fujiwara Y, Shinkai H, Yohida D, Suzuki T, Yukawa H, Yasumura S, Haga H (2003) Effects of dietary variety on declines in high-level functional capacity in elderly people living in a community. Jpn J Public Health 50:1117–1124

Chapter 5
Case Study 2 (A Prefectural Government City)

Abstract In this chapter, we verify the existence of urban food desert issues (FDs) and analyse their conditions. The case study area is the centre of prefectural government city. Many elderly people with a high risk of malnutrition live near the central shopping street. This area is close to grocery stores, and there seemed to be adequate access to food. We analysed the main factors that worsen the eating habits of the elderly people. As a result, not only their personal attributes (such as degree of independence, sex, etc.) but also social factors (factors related to local social capital such as daily habits—eating meals with others, joining local activities) are also very important. Then, we classified 57 neighbourhood associations according to the above factors and extracted five clusters. Among these five clusters, two were characterized by the poor eating habits of elderly residents. We classified these two types as food deserts. These clusters are mainly located in city centre. The above research indicates that urban-type food deserts exist in the centre of this city, and social capital is a very important cause.

Keywords Urban food deserts · A prefectural government city · Ties with neighbours · Social capital · New food desert map

5.1 Introduction

5.1.1 The Purpose of This Chapter

In this study, we verify the existence of urban food deserts (FDs) and analyse their conditions. The case study area is the centre of prefectural government City C. The discussion in this chapter is based on extensive surveys of and interviews with local residents. We clarify specifically 'who suffers from urban food desert issues, where these people live and what kind of problems they have'. The purposes of the research are as follows:

(1) An examination of elderly people's living environments in the centre of prefectural government City C.

© The Author(s), under exclusive license to Springer Nature Singapore Pte Ltd. 2021   95
N. Iwama et al., *Urban Food Deserts in Japan*, International Perspectives
in Geography 15, https://doi.org/10.1007/978-981-16-0893-3_5

(2)   The identification of areas where many elderly people with poor eating habits live.
(3)   An analysis of the factors that disrupt the dictary habits of elderly people (the verification of the existence of FDs). (Sects. 2.2–4.4. Source: Iwama et al. [2015]).
(4)   The geography of FD areas and clarification of their characteristics (Sects. 5.1–5.3. Source: Iwama et al. [2016]).

5.1.2   Outline of This Chapter

This chapter has six sections. Section 5.2 describes the survey method. Section 5.3 provides a general description of City C. This section also explains the individual attributes of elderly people and their living environments (this section corresponds to purpose 1) and is based on an analysis of the questionnaire. We ascertain the areas where many elderly people with poor eating habits live (this section corresponds to purpose 2). In Sect. 5.4, we analyse the individual attributes and living environments that disrupt dietary habits in elderly people. These individual attributes include sex, age and degree of independence. The living environment variables are 'access to food'[1] and 'ties with families and neighbours' (local social capital).[2] To analyse the relationship between these variables and elderly people's eating habits, we clarify the factors that disrupt dietary habits in elderly people (this section corresponds to purpose 3). Then, in Sect. 5.5, we classify the basic district units (neighbourhood associations[3]) of this city into groups using multivariate analysis. The variables used in this analysis are elderly people's eating habits and living environments. Then, we chose groups that have the typical characteristics of food deserts (this section corresponds to purpose 4). Finally, in Sect. 5.6, we organize the information gathered in this study.

5.2   The Survey Method

5.2.1   The Process of the Survey

The process of the survery is as follow. First, we collected documents that are necessary for understanding the outline of city C, then we studied in field. Second, we measured food access in this city by GIS (Geographical Information System). Third, we did questionnaire survey to all residents who live in city center. The questions are about their individual attitude (sex, age, family structure, where they go outside by themselves or not,[4] utilization of private car), shopping behavior (who usually go shopping, the frequency of shopping, transfer, the utilization of food delivery services, the utilization of meal delivery services, the frequency of eat canned foods and frozen foods, and what they feel uncomfortable when they go shopping), and ties with families and neighbors (the frequency of join local clubs and activities, do they eat daily meal with someone or eat alone,[5] the frequency of joining mess). Moreover, to complement questionnaire survey, we did interview surveys with many elder residents. Fourth, by simple analysis of questionnaire survey, we outlined old people's individual attitudes and their shopping behaviors. Fifth, we made a map which shows the high densely inhabited of poor eating elderly. The base unit of this map is neighbourhood associations. Then, we analyzed the special characteristics of these elderly's distribution pattern. Sixth, we carried out multilevel analysis. The dependent variable is individual dietary diversity score. The independent variables are independent attribute, food access, and the ties with families and local communities (the details are to be mentioned later). Then, we clarified the main factors that disrupt dietary habits in old people.

5.2.2 The Food Diversity Investigation

The food diversity investigation measures old people's malnutrition risks and this investigation is often used in medical science and nutrition science (more detail, please see Chap. 4, Sect. 4.1). The food diversity investigation concerned the frequency of consumption of 10 food groups (meat, fish and shellfish, eggs, milk, processed soy products, deep yellow vegetables, seaweed, fruit, potatoes, and oil and fat). Respondents were asked to indicate how often they ate each food listed above, on the following scale: (1) almost every day; (2) every other day; (3) once or twice a week; or (4) almost never. The number of "almost every day" responses is the dietary diversity score. People with low dietary diversity scores (less than 4) have a very high probability of developing a poor nutritional condition in the near future. A food diversity investigation is a useful index by which to measure the healthy eating habits of seniors.

5.2.3 The Outline of Questionnaire Survey

This research was based on "the revitalization of shopping districts promotion research project in 2012". This project was managed by X prefectural government and the government office asked us to carry out the survey of this matter in city C. We conducted the questionnaire survey in the city with the full support of the local government and local merchants association. The respondents were all householders (from 4663 households) belonging to 57 communities in the center of City C. Hard copies of the questionnaire were distributed and collected by hand by board members in each community. The investigation period was from September 2012 to January 2013, and the survey response rate was 36.4%.

5.3 The Living Environments of Old People in City Center of City C

5.3.1 The Outline of the City

City C is a prefectural capital city, located on the outskirts of the Greater Tokyo Area, with a population of about 510,000 (Population Census 2010) (Photo 5.1). From the 1960s to the 1980s, there were many individual stores and eight large retailers (including two department stores) located in the central shopping streets of the city (Photo 5.2), and indeed it used to be a regional central shopping district in the northern Greater Tokyo Area. However, because of the suburbanization of commercial functions, the number of supermarkets in the suburbs increased (Photo 5.3) and the main commercial district has lost many businesses since the 1990s (Fig. 5.1). As a result, there are few perishable food stores in the centre of City C. On the other hand, city centre has been developed. Highrise condominiums are being build and the populations of higher-income households are increasing (Photo 5.4). However, there are also many low-storied multi-dwelling houses in city centre and many low-income aged people have loved there (Photo 5.5).

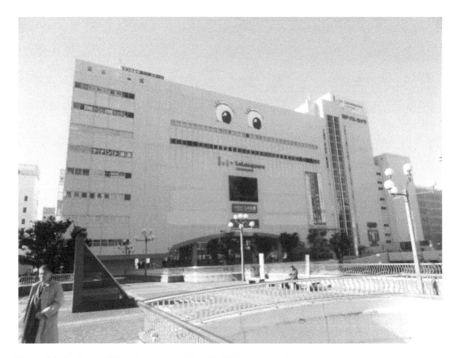

Photo 5.1 In front of C train station (City C, 2014 taken by Iwama)

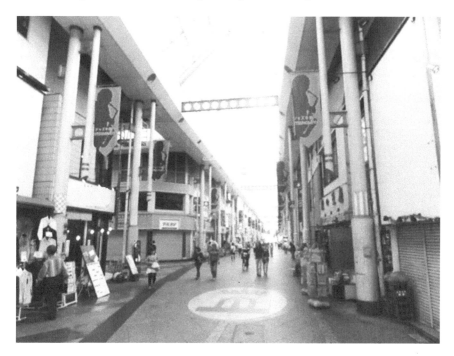

Photo 5.2 The central shopping street (City C, 2014, taken by Iwama)

5.3.2   Food Access Analysis

As noted, we cannot specify the FD area completely using geographical factors alone. However, by utilizing GIS and regional statistical data, it is possible to identify the high-risk area for FDs according to geographical factors. Figure 5.1 shows the balance of food demand (the population of old people) and food supply (the location of grocery stores and the number of visitors) (Tanaka and Komaki 2012). The kernel density estimate method can measure the surfaces (density) of supply and the surfaces of demand (Silverman 1986) (more detail, please see Chap. 3, Sect. 3.1). When we overlay these two surfaces, some areas may show a mismatch; the location where demand by far surpasses supply must be a food poverty area (the heavily shaded are in Fig. 5.1). We used the number of visitors, which is predicted from store size, as the weight to calculate the surface of supply. The population of seniors was used as the weight to calculate the surface of demand. As a smoothing parameter (or bandwidth), we used walking distance. The threshold walking distance varies according to the destination of the area or respondent. The respondents to this survey were elderly people. Koyano et al. (1991) reported that the standard distance that healthy elderly people can walk comfortably is 1 km (500 m each way); we therefore used 500 m as a parameter (Koyano et al. 1991).

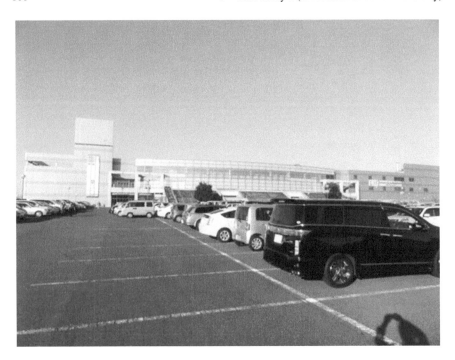

Photo 5.3   Supermarket in suburbs (City C, 2014, taken by Iwama)

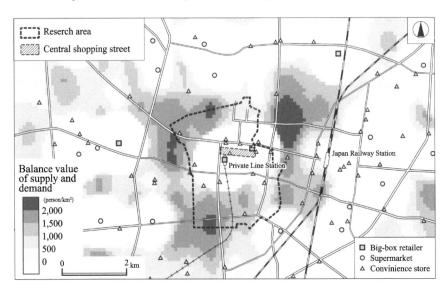

Fig. 5.1   Food access map of City C in 2010. *Source* Iwama et al. (2015, 2016)

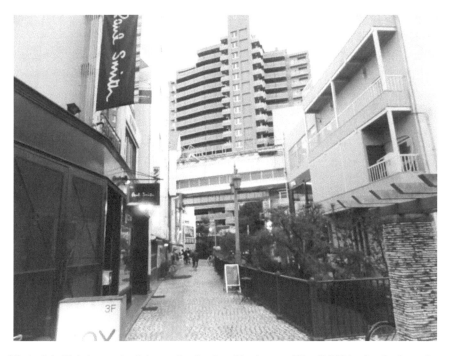

Photo 5.4 Highrise condominium and redeveloped back street (City C, 2014, taken by Iwama)

As Fig. 5.1 indicates, there is sufficient food supply (light or no shaded) in the downtown area where the main commercial district and large stores are concentrated. However, we find that food demand is much greater than food supply in the surrounding area (heavy shading), and is especially poor in the northern and southern parts of the study area. However, we should note that stores in areas with sufficient food supply are mostly convenience stores, where the food repertoire is smaller than that of food supermarkets, which sell many inexpensive fresh foods. Therefore, we consider that the shopping convenience of residents in the study area varies according to their individual circumstances.

5.3.3 Questionnaire Responses and Map of Low Dietary Diversity Scores

Next, we consider the living environment of residents as revealed by questionnaire responses. Table 5.1 shows respondents' gender, age, whether they go out alone, the presence of family members and whether they drive a private car. Most respondents were in the 60–70 s age group, with a majority of females (65.8%). We note that 85.5% of respondents had sufficient independence to go out alone by vehicle. In terms of family structure, 39.6% of residents lived with their children, while single-person households accounted for 22.1%. The proportion of respondents who drove

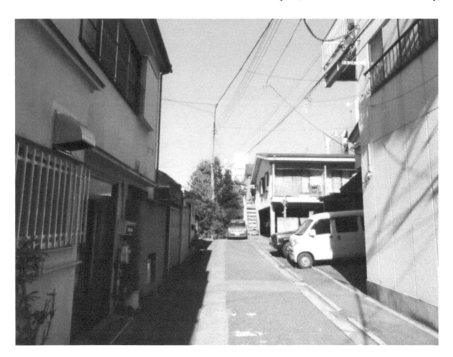

Photo 5.5 Low-storied multi-dwelling houses (City C, 2014, taken by Iwama)

a car themselves or who were driven by family members was more than 70% of the total.

Figure 5.2 shows the percentage of single elderly households by community: 25.8% are concentrated in areas around the private railway station where there is prefectural housing and low-rise apartment houses; areas with 20.5–25.7% of elderly households are located in northern areas around the prefectural office and in southern areas near City Hall. However, we find no geographical clusters on a regional scale.

Table 5.2 indicates that 62.3% of residents do their own shopping. The highest frequency of shopping per week is 3–4 times (36.9%), followed by 1–2 times (28.9%). In terms of mode of transportation to stores, walking accounts for 31.3% of respondents, bicycle 26.3%, car (self-driven) 23.7% and car (driven by a family member) 15.5%. Most respondents answered that they could access a store less than 30 min away on foot or by car. The most commonly used type of grocery store was a supermarket in the downtown area (28.8%), followed by department stores (18.3%). The proportion of respondents who made purchases at suburban supermarkets was 49.8% of the total. Few people bought food from small local shops: 11.1% purchased food on a shopping street and 24.7% used convenience stores. Furthermore, 15.0% of respondents used co-operative stores and 7.3% used the meals-on-wheels service (Table 5.3). Approximately 60% of the respondents bought frozen food.

In terms of categories of shopping problems, "difficulty in carrying purchases" was reported by 53.2% of respondents, "have no easy access to stores" by 26.9%,

Table 5.1 Individual attributes (%)

Gender		Age composition		Go out alone by private car or public transportation		Presence of family members		Whether they drive a private car	
Male	34.2	60–69	34.5	Yes	85.5	Single-person	22.1	No	22.7
Female	65.8	70–79	36.2	No	14.5	Couple	31.4	Drive a car themselves	47.0
		80–89	24.6			Living with their children	39.6	Driven by family partner	12.5
		90–99	1.9			Others	4.8	Driven by family members	15.7
		Others	1.8					Others	2.0
$n = 1,306$		$n = 1,669$		$n = 1,671$		$n = 1,671$		$n = 1,645$	

Source Iwama et al. (2015)

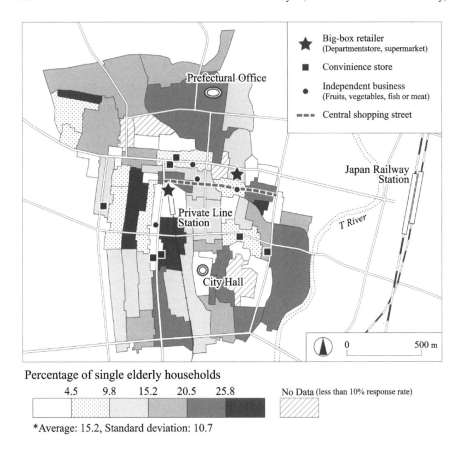

Percentage of single elderly households

4.5   9.8   15.2   20.5   25.8   No Data (less than 10% response rate)

*Average: 15.2, Standard deviation: 10.7

Fig. 5.2 Percentage of single elderly households in 2013. *Source* Iwama et al. (2015)

"concerned about diet" by 6.2%, "expense" by 3.6%, "difficulty in making purchases on rainy days" by 3.3%, and "feel uneasy about future shopping environment" by 2.2% (Table 5.4). These results show that although the residents of the study area took a great interest in the convenience of shopping for food, they did not take much interest in their diet.

Table 5.5 shows the proportion of low dietary diversity scores. Those that fall short of the standard (4 points) account for 48.9% of the total. The average dietary diversity score is 3.7, that is, just below the standard, which indicates that roughly half of old people respondents are at high risk of malnutrition. The male ratio of low dietary diversity scores is higher than that of females.

As people grow older, they generally prefer a healthy and simple diet. In Japan, females usually have more cooking experience and tend to have healthier eating behaviours than males. In many families, it is usually the wife who makes family meals. Japanese females usually also live much longer than Japanese males. If a female loses her partner and becomes isolated from society, her motivation for healthy

Table 5.2 Shopping activities (%)

Residents who do their own shopping		Frequency of shopping per week		Modes of transportation to stores		Time required from their houses to stores (self-enumeration)		Stores in which they usually purchase daily foods			Sometimes use stores on shopping streets	Sometimes use convenience sotes
								Main stores				
Themselves	62.3	Everyday	16.6	On foot	31.3	Less than 10 min	26.9	Downtown area			11.1	24.7
Partners	26.5	5–6 times	15.2	Bicycle	26.3	10–15 min	35.7	Department store	18			
Their children	8.9	3–4 times	36.9	Bus	1.4	15–30 min	32.1	Supermarket	29			
Caretaker	0.7	1–2 times	28.9	Car (self-driven)	23.7	30–60 min	4.7	Suburb				
Others	1.6	Few times per month	2.4			More than 60 min	0.6	Supermarkets (plu.)	49.8			
				Car (driven by family member)	15.5			Others	3.1			
				Others	1.7							
n = 1,645		n = 1,613		n = 1,618		n = 658						n = 1,397

Source Iwama et al. (2015)

Table 5.3 Usage of food delivery service (%)

Home-delivery service		Meals-on-wheels service		Frequency of eat frozen foods or canned foods	
Already use	15.0	Already use	7.3	Almost everyday	1.5
Plan to use	7.6	Plan to use	8.2	Once every two days	9.8
No use	77.4	No use	84.5	Sometimes	46.7
				No	41.9
$n = 1,569$		$n = 1,600$		$n = 775$	

Source Iwama et al. (2015)

Table 5.4 Shopping problems

	(%)
Difficulty in carrying purchases	53.2
No easy access to stores	26.9
Concerned about diet	6.2
Expense	3.6
Difficulty in making purchases on rainy days	3.3
Feel uneasy about future shopping Environment	2.2
Lack of car parking	1.2
Difficulty in shopping at large scale stores	0.9
Others	2.5
	$n = 769$

Source Iwama et al. (2015)

cooking tends to decrease. Thus, strength is decreased not only by aging, but by a loss of motivation through isolation that leads to a rapid decrease in the dietary diversity scores of females over 90 years old.

Figure 5.3 shows a map of the percentages of elderly respondents with low dietary diversity scores (i.e. at high risk of malnutrition). It is evident that old people who have a poor diet live in the downtown area.

5.4 Analysis of Factors That Disrupt Healthy Eating Habits

5.4.1 Analysis Procedures

In this section, obstacles to healthy eating are analysed quantitatively using multilevel analysis. The dependent variable is individual dietary diversity scores. The analysis is performed using two direct effects models (models 1 and 2) and three interaction models (models 3, 4 and 5).

Table 5.5 Food diversity scores (by gender and age)

Age composition	Elderly people with diversity scores over 4 (%)	Elderly people with diversity scores less than 4 (%)
Male		
60–69	36.7	63.3
70–79	44.2	55.8
80–89	57.0	43.0
90–99	57.1	42.9
Total	43.4	56.6
Female		
60–69	57.1	42.9
70–79	52.8	47.2
80–89	53.4	46.6
90–99	23.1	76.9
Total	54.1	45.9
Total	51.1	48.9
The average of dietary diversity scores		3.7
		$n = 1{,}639$

Source Iwama et al. (2015)

The independent variables are "gender", "age", "going out alone", "participating in events" and "eating meals with someone else", from which nonstandard partial regression coefficients are calculated at the individual and group levels (community level) in model 1. "Presence of supermarket" is added to the above independent variables at the group level in model 2.

The interaction effects between "presence of supermarket" (a group-level variable) and individual-level variables are examined in the interaction models. To examine these effects, the following are used as individual-level variables in these models: "going out alone" in model 3, "participating in events" in model 4 and "eating meals with someone else" in model 5.

5.4.2 Direct Effects Model

Table 5.6 shows the analysis results for model 1. All individual-level independent variables are statistically significant at the 5% level. From the nonstandard partial regression coefficients, people with high dietary diversity scores are elderly females who frequently go out, participate in events and eat meals with someone else. In contrast, the "age" and "going out alone" variables are statistically significant at the 5% level at the group level. These results mean that dietary diversity scores are higher in communities with a higher average age or with larger proportions of people

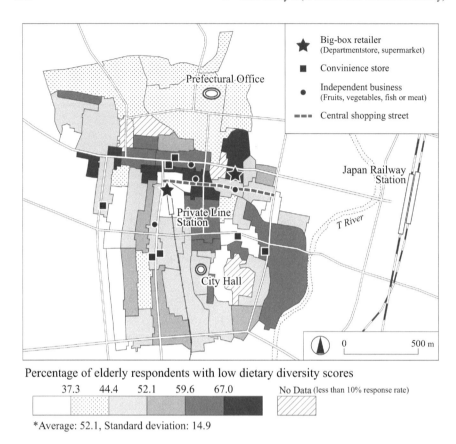

Percentage of elderly respondents with low dietary diversity scores

37.3   44.4   52.1   59.6   67.0   No Data (less than 10% response rate)

*Average: 52.1, Standard deviation: 14.9

Fig. 5.3 Percentage of elderly respondents with low dietary diversity scores in 2013. *Source* Iwama et al. (2015)

who frequently go out alone. The trend for dietary diversity scores to be lower in communities with a higher proportion of men is statistically significant at the 10% level.

The results of model 2 are shown in Table 5.6. The individual-level results are almost the same as those in model 1. The variables of "age" and "going out alone" are statistically significant at the group level, while "presence of supermarket" is not. A trend is seen in the dietary diversity scores of people who frequently eat with someone else to be higher than those of people who do not, because "eating meals with someone else" is statistically significant at the 10% level. The adaptability of model 2 is slightly higher than that of model 1; Akaike's information criterion (AIC) (an index showing the adaptability of a model) is 4975.2 in model 1 and 4972.2 in model 2.

Table 5.6 Result of multilevel analysis: direct effect model

	Model 1		Model 2	
	Partial regression coefficient	p-value	Partial regression coefficient	p-value
Individual level				
Gender (Ref.: Male)	−0.783	0.000	−0.783	0.000
Age	0.319	0.001	0.319	0.001
Going out alone	0.666	0.011	0.666	0.011
Participating in event	0.313	0.000	0.313	0.000
Taking a meal with someone	0.299	0.000	0.299	0.000
Group level				
Gender (Ref.: Male)	−0.938	0.060	−0.791	0.115
Age	1.127	0.012	1.051	0.033
Going out alone	2.442	0.002	2.423	0.004
Participating in event	−0.119	0.725	−0.051	0.883
Taking a meal with someone	0.396	0.104	0.438	0.066
Presence of supermarket (Ref.: Yes)	–	–	−0.146	0.378
AIC	4975.229		4972.245	

Source Iwama et al. (2015)

5.4.3 Interaction Model

Table 5.7 shows the results from the interaction model. Model 3 examines the interaction effect between "presence of supermarket" at the group level and "going out alone" at the individual level. "Going out alone" at the individual level is statistically significant at the 10% level, while "presence of supermarket" at the group level is not, which means that "going out alone" improves residents' dietary diversity score to a greater extent in communities with a supermarket than in those without.

"Presence of supermarket" at the group level is not statistically significant in model 4, which examines its interaction effect with "participating in events". The interaction effect between "presence of supermarket" at the group level and "participating in events" at the individual level is not statistically significant.

Likewise, in model 5, which examines its interaction effect with "taking a meal with someone", the interaction effect between "presence of supermarket" at the group level and "taking a meal with someone" at the individual level is not statistically significant. "Presence of supermarket" at the group level is not statistically significant. As noted above, comparison of AIC indices of the models shows that adaptability is highest in model 3.

Table 5.7 Results from the interaction model

	Model 3		Model 4		Model 5	
	Partial regression coefficient	p-value	Partial regression coefficient	p-value	Partial regression coefficient	p-value
Individual level						
Gender (Ref.: Male)	−0.781	0.000	−0.777	0.000	−0.781	0.000
Age	0.317	0.001	0.320	0.001	0.312	0.001
Participating in event	0.304	0.000	–	–	0.307	0.000
Taking a meal with someone	0.303	0.000	0.300	0.000	–	–
Going out alone	–	–	0.665	0.012	0.660	0.013
Presence of supermarket (Ref.: Yes)	–	–	–	–	–	–
Presence of supermarket × Going out alone	−5.653	0.088	–	–	–	–
Presence of supermarket × Participating in event	–	–	−0.226	0.511	–	–
Presence of supermarket × Taking a meal with someone	–	–	–	–	−0.336	0.279
Group level						
Gender (Ref.: Male)	−0.791	0.115	−0.791	0.114	−0.792	0.114
Age	1.051	0.033	1.051	0.033	1.051	0.033
Participating in event	−0.049	0.883	−0.051	0.883	−0.051	0.883
Taking a meal with someone	0.439	0.066	0.438	0.065	0.438	0.065
Going out alone	2.426	0.004	2.423	0.004	2.423	0.004
Presence of supermarket (Ref.: Yes)	−0.146	0.378	−0.146	0.377	−0.146	0.377
AIC	4969.786		4976.087		4974.986	

Source Iwama et al. (2015)

5.4.4 Summary of Multilevel Analysis

Figure 5.3 indicates that the areas in City A where old people have poor eating habits are located in the downtown area near the main shopping street. Figure 5.1 illustrates food access, but cannot explain why the living environment in the downtown area is worse despite the number of grocery stores being relatively high. As expected, we believe that food access in the downtown area affects the residents' diet.

Moreover, we cannot find a geographical correlation between the distribution of single-person households (Fig. 5.2) and households with low dietary diversity scores (Fig. 5.2). We conducted geographically weighted regression analyses using the percentage of elderly people with low dietary diversity scores as a dependent variable and the percentage of single elderly householders in each community as the independent variable. The adjusted coefficient of determination (r2) was 0.036, which shows that there is a poor geographical correlation between the two variables. These results indicate the relevance of other influential factors in addition to individual factors, such as whether the householder lives alone.

The findings from the multilevel analyses can be summarized as follows. When there is no difference between the characteristics of communities according to the control variables, the individuals with a high dietary diversity score are elderly females who regularly go out, participate in events and eat meals with someone else.

The results of analysis by community show that communities with high dietary diversity scores are characterized by residents with a high average age, who go out frequently, and eat meals with others. In addition, diet diversity scores tend to be high in a community with a high proportion of people who go out frequently when there is no supermarket in the area.

The results of these analyses mean that for the elderly persons with low degree of independence, the malnutrition risk is higher in the area without nearby grocery stores than in the are with nearby grocery stores. In short, the results of these analyses indicate that the eating behaviours of seniors are severely affected by not only individual attributes and age, but also by social ties with neighbours and family (whether they often participate in community events or eat with others). These results suggest that it is possible to make FD maps using factors of food access and social capital. Therefore, in the next section, we try to make FD map in city C.

5.5 The Geography of FD Areas and Their Characteristics

5.5.1 The Survey Method

We classified 57 neighbourhood associations into groups using multivariate analysis. The variables in this analysis are elderly people's eating habits and living environments. To perform a multivariate analysis, we must check the correlations among the variables and carefully select those to be used in this analysis. Therefore, we first constructed a database showing the following eight variables according to the neighbourhood association. We then performed a principal component analysis using this database. Second, we extracted the variables from the principal component analysis and used them to perform a cluster analysis.

The analysis in Sect. 5.4 shows that individual attributes (especially 'degree of independence'), ties with families and neighbours, and access to food have a strong influence on urban food deserts. In addition, eating habits (the 'investigation of food diversity' score) are also an important factor that reveals the degree of disadvantage to the aged inhabitants caused by urban food deserts. In addition, age and sex have strong influences on the eating habits of elderly people, but these factors have a strong correlation with the degree of independence. Therefore, we did not use age and sex in this analysis. We used the following eight variables in principal component analysis: *Degree of independence* (1. whether elderly people can travel by private car or public transportation: 'going out'); *access to food* (2. whether there is a grocery store within 500 m of their houses: 'store within 500 m'); *ties to families and neighbours* (3. The percentage of elderly people who usually dine with someone else: 'dine together'); 4. The percentage of elderly people who sometimes dine with someone else: 'sometimes dine together'[6]; 5. The percentage of single families: 'proportion living alone'; 6. the percentage of elderly people who organize local events by themselves: 'event organization'; 7. the percentage of elderly people who actively participate in local events positively 'active event participation',[7] and *eating habits* (8. the percentage of elderly people whose food diversity investigation scores are lower than 3: 'low food diversity score').

5.5.2   The Grouping of the Neighbourhood Associations

The principal component analysis produced three main components (Table 5.8). The primary component shows a high loading on 'dine together' and 'going out' and high negative loadings on 'proportion living alone' and 'low food diversity score'. The second principal component shows a high loading on 'store within 500 m', 'sometimes dine together' and 'event organization'. The third component shows a relatively high loading on 'active event participation'.

The primary component is ties with family. This component suggests that in the neighbourhood associations where many people live with their families, people tend to dine with someone else, maintain a high degree of independence and maintain good eating habits. The second component is ties with the local community. This component suggests that in the neighbourhood associations where many community leaders live, regardless of the family component, people tend to dine with others. In addition, these districts also tend to have good shopping environments. The third component is the number of people who actively participate in local events.

Next, to examine the characteristics of the neighbourhood associations, we employed a KS-means cluster analysis. (Asakawa 2008). It is widely known that

Table 5.8 Result of principal component analysis

	The primary component	The second component	The third component
Dine together	0.844	−0.165	0.160
Proportion living alone	−0.769	−0.234	−0.182
Going out	0.752	0.179	−0.329
Low food diversity score	−0.485	0.287	0.457
Store within 500 m	0.284	0.692	−0.113
Sometimes dine together	−0.244	0.684	0.119
Event organization	−0.121	0.663	−0.205
Active event participation	0.278	0.053	0.830
Characteristic value	2.3	1.6	1.1
Contribution ratio	29.2	19.8	14.2
Cumulative contribution ratio	29.2	49.0	63.2

Source Iwama et al. (2016)

the results of such analyses are strongly affected by the variables used. Four variables had high positive and negative loadings on the primary component, and three had high loadings on the second component. Therefore, we deleted 'going out' from the primary component and evened the number of variables between the primary and the second components.[8] Note that 'going out' is the variable that shows elderly people's degree of independence. Degree of independence is not directly connected to the living environment. Therefore, we considered that 'going out' is less important than the other three variables in this analysis. In addition, we can achieve our research goals using the primary and secondary components.[9] We deleted 'active event participation', which belonged to the third component.[10] Therefore, we narrowed the variables down to six and conducted the KS-method cluster analysis using these six variables.

As a result, 57 neighbourhood associations were classified into five clusters (Table 5.9). In cluster A, there are many grocery stores, few single households, many people who dine with someone else, and many leaders of local events. The percentage of elderly people categorized as having a high risk of malnutrition (with food diversity scores of less than three) was 42.0%, which was the lowest percentage among the clusters. Therefore, we named districts in cluster A the 'Low-risk districts'. In cluster B there were relatively few grocery stores. However, many people dined

Table 5.9 Characteristics of each cluster

		Proportion living alone	Event organization	Dine together	Sometimes dine together	Low food diversity score	Store within 500 m
Cluster A	Low-risk districts	15.0	5.4	64.9	13.0	42.0	1.0
Cluster B	Risk-free districts	20.0	4.8	64.6	7.1	48.1	0.6
Cluster C	Potentially high-risk districts	25.9	2.5	59.6	10.8	50.1	0.1
Cluster D	Moderate-risk districts	28.8	3.0	50.8	5.8	54.3	0.3
Cluster E	High-risk districts	21.6	1.2	55.3	20.8	58.3	1.0

Source Iwama et al. (2016)

with someone else and the percentage of elderly people at high risk of malnutrition was relatively low (48.1%). Therefore, we named districts in cluster B the 'Risk-free districts'. In cluster C there were few grocery stores and the percentage of single households was high. The percentage of elderly people with a high risk of malnutrition was 50.1%. We named districts in cluster C the 'Potentially high-risk districts'. Cluster D has the following characteristics: a high percentage of single households, a high percentage of people eating alone, and few neighbourhood grocery stores. We named districts in this cluster the 'Moderate-risk districts'. Cluster E has the following characteristics: a high percentage of elderly people with a high risk of malnutrition, good access to food, few local leaders to organize community events, and a relatively high percentage of people eating alone. We named districts in this cluster the 'High-risk districts'.

5.5.3   The Characteristics of Each Cluster and the Identification of Food Desert Districts

5.5.3.1   The Characteristics of the Clusters

Figure 5.4 shows the locations of the above clusters. The high-risk districts are mainly located in the city centre. There are many offices and retail stores in the city centre, but relatively few residential areas. This district has a mixture of high-rise upmarket condominiums (which are mainly located in redeveloped areas) and a zone of low-rise wooden houses (located in old residential areas). On the other hand, moderate-risk districts and potentially high-risk districts are located on the fringes of central urban areas. Risk-free districts are separated and there are few geographical

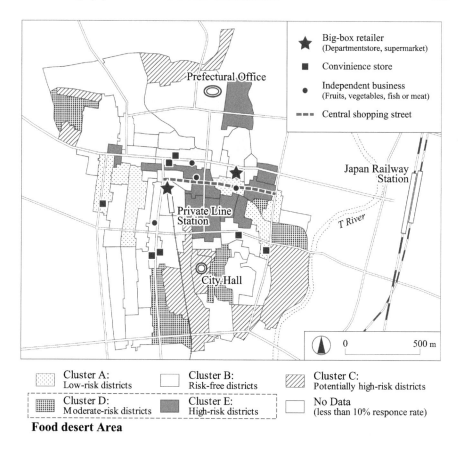

Fig. 5.4 Locations of the clusters in 2013 (Food desert map). *Source* Iwama et al. (2016)

location patterns. Low-risk districts were located in parts of the city centre such as north-west of the city hall and west of the private railway station. These areas are known as the upper socioeconomic residential areas of City C.

The clusters can be summarized as follows. A high-risk district is a cluster with the highest percentages of elderly people with a high risk of malnutrition. Districts in this cluster are mainly located in areas with many offices and stores. The night-time population of these areas is small compared with other districts. In addition, the number of migrants (people moving in or out) is considerable. Ties within the local community are generally weak. The percentage of the population aged 65 or older and proportion of single households are high. Therefore, it seems that many elderly residents are isolated from local society in these districts.

Moderate-risk districts are those with the second highest risk of malnutrition for elderly people. This cluster's characteristics are poor access to food (few neighbourhood grocery stores) and relatively weak ties with families and local communities. Moreover, there are many single-person households. These facts mean that it is very difficult for elderly people to shop because of the lack of neighbourhood grocery stores and the lack of support from family members and neighbours.

Potentially high-risk districts also have a relatively high risk of malnutrition. The access to food in these districts is as poor as that in moderate-risk districts. However, people in these districts maintain relatively good relationships with family and neighbours. Therefore, compared with the elderly in moderate-risk districts, elderly residents can receive help with shopping from their family members and neighbours.

Risk-free districts have relatively good food diversity scores. It seems that many elderly people live with their children and they have good relations with their neighbours. Therefore, although some areas have low access to food, many people support the elderly (helping with shopping, sharing meals, etc.) and the residents overcome their poor living environment (low access to food) through strong local mutual aid.[11] Therefore, the elderly people of these districts generally maintain healthy eating habits.

'Low-risk districts' show the healthiest eating habits among elderly residents. These districts have good shopping environments. In addition, many elderly people live with their families and the local communities are generally active. This cluster includes many upmarket residential districts.

5.5.3.2   The Geography of FD Areas

In the above analyses, we concluded that the food desert areas of City C are the high- and moderate-risk districts, which we show in Fig. 5.4. Therefore, Fig. 5.4 is the new food desert map showing both a special factor (access to food) and a social factor (social capital). Figure 5.5 shows the characteristics of each cluster based on food access and SC. This map indicates the two characteristics of food deserts. They are: (1) areas where local social capital is very low, and the living environment of elderly people has deteriorated because of the lack of mutual assistance by neighbours and family members (high-risk districts), and (2) access to food and social capital are relatively poor, which induces deterioration in elderly people's living environments (high-risk districts). The former type of food desert can be found in the centre of large cities, and the latter type is common on the fringes of cities. Our research also suggests that conditions in food deserts of type 1) are more serious than those prevailing in type 2).

Previously, mainstream food desert studies have been spatial analyses mainly concerned with food deserts of type 2) (the blank areas in maps showing grocery stores). However, we conducted an analysis of the social factors of urban food deserts on a micro-scale. This research found a new type of food desert, type 1). The characteristics of types 1) and 2) are very different. The problem in type 2) food deserts

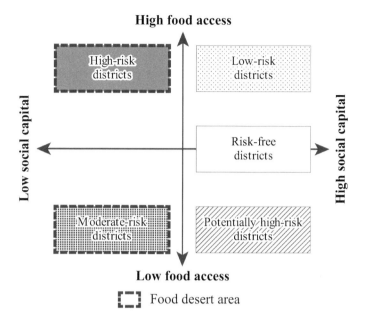

Fig. 5.5 Characteristics of local communities based on food access and social capital. *Source* Iwama et al. (2016)

is the lack of neighbourhood grocery stores, so improving access to food is the top priority in such cases. On the other hand, in cases of type 1), the problem is isolation from families and local society. Many of the elderly people who live in type 1) districts have lost the motivation to maintain a healthy lifestyle and eating habits. In such areas, the revitalization of social ties must be the most important policy to improve living conditions.

This research has also pointed out the following two facts. First, living environments are very different even within a city centre. Therefore, we must analyse food desert issues on a micro-scale (such as neighbourhood associations). Second, as Tables 5.4 and 5.5 show, many residents are at high risk of malnutrition but do not realize it.

5.6 Summary of This Chapter

In this study, we verify the existence of urban food deserts and analyse their conditions. The case study area is the centre of prefectural government City C. In this chapter, we clarified the following points.

The centre of City C used to have one of the largest shopping streets. Not only locals but also people from the outskirts of this city or from other prefectures enjoyed shopping there. However, the number of grocery stores is decreasing in the city centre and many large supermarkets have opened on the outskirts of City C. Therefore, there are areas with poor access to food in the northern and southern districts of the city centre. However, many residents shop in the suburbs, travelling by car or bicycle and find no difficulty in obtaining food.

Many elderly people with a high risk of malnutrition live near the central shopping street. This area is close to grocery stores, and there seemed to be adequate access to food. Therefore, no one had paid any attention to this area, which was a blind spot and there was no support programme for these elderly people from the local government. There are few elderly people in single-person households, so living environment factors other than poor access to food and single households have a strong influence on the eating habits of elderly people in this area.

We analysed the main factors that worsen the eating habits of the elderly people. As a result, not only their personal attributes (such as degree of independence, sex, etc.) but also local factors (factors related to local social capital such as daily habits—eating meals with others, joining local activities) are also very important. On the other hand, the influence of the shopping environment (access to food) was limited. These facts suggest that in the centre of City C there are food deserts caused by the decline of local social capital.

We classified 57 neighbourhood associations according to the above factors and extracted five clusters. Among these five clusters, two were characterized by the poor eating habits of elderly residents. We classified these two types as food deserts. The first type of cluster is comprised of neighbourhood associations with good access to food, but local social capital is quite low and many elderly people are isolated from their families and neighbours. In these areas, many elderly people are unable to obtain sufficient support from families and neighbours or have lost their motivation to maintain healthy eating habits. Therefore, although they live in convenient shopping environments, their eating habits are generally worse than those of other areas. The second cluster is comprised of neighbourhood associations with relatively poor access to food and where social capital is also relatively low. The average distance to the nearest grocery stores is 500–1000 m in this cluster. It is somewhat difficult for elderly people to go shopping every day by themselves. However, they receive little assistance from their families or neighbours. Therefore, their eating habits are worsening.

The above research indicates that urban-type food deserts exist in the centre of City C, and social capital is more important cause than food access there. The characteristics of urban and rural food deserts caused by poor access to food are totally different.

In urban food deserts, the revitalization of ties with people is more important than any shopping assistance program. Families and neighbours can have a strong influence on elderly people who stay at home, and such elderly people may go outside and improve their shopping and eating habits.[12] In addition, in areas where the residents offset elderly people's poor shopping habits by helping with shopping and sharing food with elderly people, financial support from government and large retail companies for such neighbourhood activities would produce good results and improve elderly people's eating habits.[13] We must understand the characteristics of each type of food desert and consider an appropriate response in each area.

Notes

1. The distance between their house and the nearest grocery. For more details, please see Chap. 3, Sect. 3.1
2. Social capital means (1) the social network (interpersonal ties and inter-populational ties) and (2) trust and reciprocity normative consciousness fostered by social networks. For more details, please see Chap. 3, Sect. 3.2.
3. Japanese neighbourhood associations are private organizations with the purpose of improving local living environments in co-operation with local governments. Neighbourhood associations are established based on the town street unit. Although it is not obligatory for residents to participate in the neighbourhood association, participation rates are high.
4. The measure to understand the old people's self-supported degree in their daily lives. In particular, w e ask "could you go outside by yourself using car, public buses and trains?". This measure has been widely used in Social welfare and medical sciences (Ministry of Health, Labour and Welfare 1993).
5. In this chapter, we measured the tie with families and neighbors using following two indexes; the participations of vertical and horizontal organizations (neigh-bourhood associations and local clubs such as sports activities and hobbies), and the frequency and deps of the communication among their neighbors (the existence of the person to eat meal together, the frequency of dining meal together). These indexes are categorized as "Structural social capital". These measures have been widely used by governments such as Ministry of Health, Labour and Welfare. The purpose of this research is to clarify the influence which local level factors make to old person's eating habits. Therefore, we have not calculated "Recognition social capital".
6. 'Dine together' and 'sometimes dine together' are independent factors. The former factor refers to people living with their families. In contrast, the latter factor refers to people who live alone but have strong ties with the local community. Therefore, they have many opportunities to enjoy dining with others.
7. 'Event organization' and 'active event participation' are independent factors. The former refers to altruistic behaviours such as attending to others and plan-ning/conducting social events enthusiastically. The latter refers to participating in local events planned and conducted by others. Of the two, 'event organiza-tion' is the more advanced social role. It is safe to say that 'event organization' requires the ability to act as a local leader. On the other hand, 'active event participation' indicates ties with neighbours (Lawton 1972).
8. We had to maintain a balance between the first and second principal compo-nents. Therefore, we selected the top three factors from each principal compo-nent. In the first principal component, there were four factors with high factor loadings. One of the factors was 'going out'. This factor refers to old

people's degree of independence. The degree of independence was not directly connected with old people's living environments. It is safe to say that 'going out' is less important than the other three factors. Therefore, we dropped this factor and selected three factors from the first principal component.

9. The third principal component has no strong connection with the food diversity scores and access to food. Moreover, the value of this characteristic was low (1.1), so we decided that this component was not important in this analysis.

10. 'Active event participation' has a different character from the second principal component, which refers to ties with the local community. We surmise that the people who did not connect with the local community also answered 'active event participation'.

11. Our study area is within 1 km of the central shopping street, and this area has no areas with extremely poor access to food, such as remote agricultural districts, mountains, fishing villages or disaster-stricken areas. Therefore, mutual aid between neighbours can ameliorate the study area's inconvenient shopping environments.

12. Please see Chap. 7, Sect. 7.2, case study 1.

13. Please see Chap. 7, Sect. 7.2, case study 3.

References

Asakawa T (2008) Social area analysis reconsidered: structural comparison between the Tokyo and Keihanshin metropolitan areas using the KS method of cluster analysis. Jpn Sociol Rev 234:299–315 (Japanese with English abstract)

Iwama N, Asakawa T, Tanaka K, Komaki N (2015) Analysis of the factors that disrupt dietary habits in the elderly: verification of the issue of food deserts using GIS and multilevel analysis. J Food Syst Res 22(2):55–69 (Japanese with English abstract)

Iwama N, Asakawa T, Tanaka K, Komaki N (2016) Improving food desert maps based on access to food and social capital to understand factors affecting the dietary conditions of elderly residents: Case study of the centre of a local city. E-Journal GEO 11(1):70–84 (Japanese with English abstract)

Koyano W, Shibata H, Nakazato K, Haga H, Suyama Y (1991) Measurement of competence: reliability and validity of the TMIG index of competence. Gerontol Geriatr 13(2):103-116 (Japanese with English abstract)

Lawton MP (1972) The dimensions of morale. In: Kent D, Kastenbaum R, Sherwood S (eds) Research planning and action for the elderly: the power and potential of social science. Behavioural Publications, New York, pp 144–165

Ministry of Health, Labour and Welfare (1993) The notice by the head of the department for the old people's welfare (Japanese) http://www.pref.okayama.jp/uploaded/life/57625_197430_misc. pdf. Accessed 14 Aug 2020

Population Census (2010) https://www.stat.go.jp/data/kokusei/2010/. Accessed 9 Mar 2021

Silverman BW (1986) Density estimation. Chapman and Hall, London

Tanaka K, Komaki N (2012) Statistical measurement of food deserts. ESTRELA 224:9–15 (Japanese)

Chapter 6
Case Study 3 (A Small City)

Abstract We will verify the food desert (FD) issues in a small city. This city is a satellite city in Tokyo and has two distinct districts: a residential district and an agricultural district. In addition, we assessed the mobile selling vehicle service operating in the city. We found that shopping destination blank areas are largely located in the eastern agricultural areas of this city. However, high malnutrition risk old people live not only in these poor food access agricultural areas but also in the city centres which maintains good food access. Our surveys suggest that there are two main living environmental factors which exacerbate old residents' healthy eating habits: local level social capital and food access. The mobile selling vehicle supports disadvantaged old residents' daily lives. For some old residents, this service is their lifeline. However, the vehicle stops do not fully cover high malnutrition risk elderly people's residential areas. The usage of the mobile selling vehicle is high not only in the areas where there are many old people with difficulty in going out on foot (low food access areas), but also in the areas where there are many elderly who suffer from isolation and poverty (poverty areas and low social capital areas). We should consider shopping support service again from the viewpoint of FD issues and improve this problem.

Keywords Urban food deserts · Small city · Shopping destination blank areas · Social capital · Mobile vending vehicle service

6.1 Introduction

6.1.1 Purpose of This Chapter

In this chapter, we will verify the food desert (FD) issues in small city D. City D is a satellite city in Tokyo. This city has two distinct districts: a residential district and an agricultural district. As we mentioned before, the decrease of local level social capital is one of the most significant factors for the occurrence of urban type FDs issues. City D might have two types of FD characters: urban FDs and rural FDs. In addition, we evaluate a shopping assistance program (mobile selling vehicle service) operated in this city. The research subjects are as follows.

© The Author(s), under exclusive license to Springer Nature Singapore Pte Ltd. 2021
N. Iwama et al., *Urban Food Deserts in Japan*, International Perspectives
in Geography 15, https://doi.org/10.1007/978-981-16-0893-3_6

1. To understand old people's living environment in the small city and to clarify the areas where many high-malnutrition risk people live.
2. To investigate the living environment factors that impede old people's healthy eating habits [Sects. 6.2.1–6.2.3. Source: Asakawa et al. (2016)].
3. To comprehend existing shopping support program (mobile selling vehicle service) and to evaluate it from the viewpoint of FD issues [Sects. 6.3.1–6.3.4. Source: Iwama et al. (2016)].

6.1.2 An Outline of This Chapter

This chapter is made of two sections. In Sect. 6.2, we make a map which shows the living areas of malnutrition risk old people. And then, we will research the relationships between these malnutrition risk areas and FD areas. In particular, we statistically investigate whether elderly people's healthy eating habits are defined by their living environments, such as food access and social capital. This investigation is based on an analysis of the questionnaire. In Sect. 6.3, we weigh the mobile selling vehicle's routes and its sales results against the distribution of FD areas. And then, we will evaluate the effectiveness of these shopping assistant programs.

6.1.3 The Survey Method

The analytical procedure is as follows. First, we explained the outline of City D and made a food access map of this city using GIS (Geographical Information System). Next, based on the questionnaire, we analyzed the individual attributes, such as sex, age and family construct.

Second, we conducted a questionnaire survey on old people who live in this city. The questions are about their individual attributes (sex, age, family structure, economic condition,[1] eating habits), shopping behaviour (who usually goes shopping, the frequency of shopping, transport measures to stores, the utilization of food delivery services, the utilization of meal delivery services, the frequency of eating canned foods and frozen foods, the problems which they have when they go shopping), ties with families and neighbours (the frequency of joining local clubs and activities, whether they eat their daily meals with someone or alone,[2] the frequency of dining with someone) and the food diversity investigation. Moreover, to complement the questionnaire survey, we conducted interview surveys with many elderly residents. Third, we made a map which shows the areas where many high-malnutrition risk old people live. Fourth, we analyzed the main factors which disturb old people's healthy eating habits from the perspective of individual attributes and living environments (food access and the ties with families and neighbours). In sum, we did the multivariate logistic regression. The dependent variable is the food diversity score, and the independent variables are some variables which are related to individual attributes and living environments. Fifth, we grasped the outline of the mobile selling vehicle service which is under operation in City D, and we made a map which shows the distribution of this vehicle's stops. In addition, we analyzed the number of customers and the results for sales per vehicle stop. Sixth, we compared the distribution of the residential areas of malnutrition-risk old people and the vehicle stops and discussed their consistency. Seventh, we investigated the relationship between the number of customers and each vehicle stop's geographical conditions (food access, ties with families and neighbours and the residents' individual attributes).

6.1.4 An Outline of the Questionnaire Survey

We conducted the questionnaire survey in the city with the full support of the city hall and Consumers' Co-operative (Co-op). Hard copies of the questionnaire were distributed and collected by the city hall. The questionnaire was made by us. The investigation period was from February to March of 2014. We randomly picked out 5,500 persons who were over 65 years old from this city (total population of old people in this city over 65 years old is 16,428). The survey response rate was 72.4%. The questionnaires' data are identifiable information. Therefore, the city hall has kept these documents confidential. We received the data set which the city hall had processed and deleted some personal information, such as respondents' names and addresses. We integrated this individual data to the town street unit and performed some statistical analyses. City D is made of 72 town streets.

6.1.5 The Survey of Mobile Selling Vehicle Service

We collected many kinds of data about the mobile selling vehicle service from Co-op. The data include: (1) the total number of customers who used this vehicle from the first week of February to the last week of September in 2015, (2) the total sales during the above mentioned period, (3) the total sales per items and (4) each vehicle stop's (the place where this vehicle stops and sells the items to the residents) customer numbers and total sales. These data were tallied on a daily basis.

6.1.6 An Outline of City D

City D is a small city located radius 50 km form central Tokyo. The total population is 81,684 and the per cent of old people over 65 years of age is 20.2% (the national census, 2010). Compared with the national average, the ratio of the elderly is relatively low in this city and the total population is increasing slightly. City D is a satellite city of Tokyo, and there are many housing complexes in the western area of this city (Photo 6.1). Many of the residents who live in the western housing complex are so-called "new comers" who moved to this city in the 1960s and 70s. On the other hand, the eastern side is an agricultural area and many residents there are engaged in agriculture (Photo 6.2). They are so-called "old comers" who have lived in this area for many generations.

The central shopping area is located along the main streets which run through the western area (Photo 6.3). There are 11 supermarkets and many grocery stores in the west. In the east, on the other hand, we can see few convenience stores. The increase of large-scale retailers and the decrease of individual stores are remarkable. There were 547 retailers and the total floor space was 78,202 m^2 in 1997. In 2012, the total number of retailers decreased to 346, but the total floor space was 101,046 m^2. Ten fixed-route buses operate in City D, but many of them operate only in the western area.

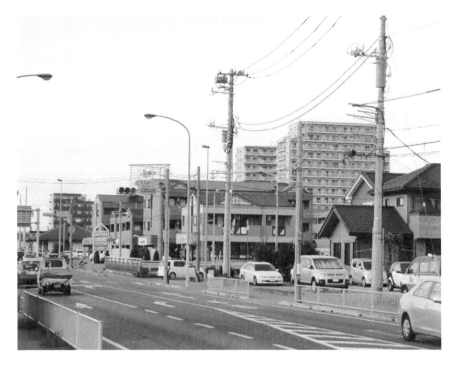

Photo 6.1 Housing complexes in the western area (City D, 2015, taken by Iwama)

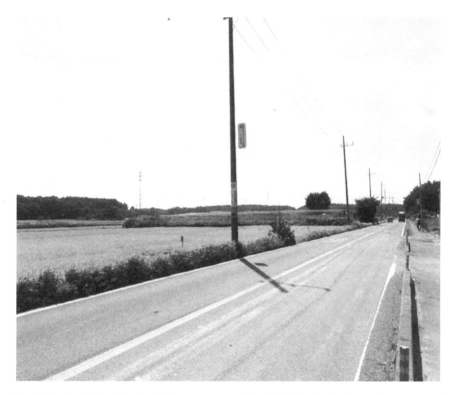

Photo 6.2 Agricultural districts in the eastern area (City D, 2015, taken by Iwama)

6.1.7 Food Access

Figure 6.1 shows the accessibility to the nearest grocery store. The ashy colour area means that the food access is low there and shopping is difficult for the residents without private cars. This figure suggests that there are many shopping destination blank areas in the west.

6.2 The Factors Which Impede Old People's Healthy Eating Habits

To prove clearly the hypothesis that living environments impede old people's healthy eating habits (i.e., to prove the existence of FDs), we conducted statistical analyses using the questionnaire data mentioned above. If old people's eating habits have clear correlations with living environments, such as food access and local level social capital, it suggests that FDs exist in this city.

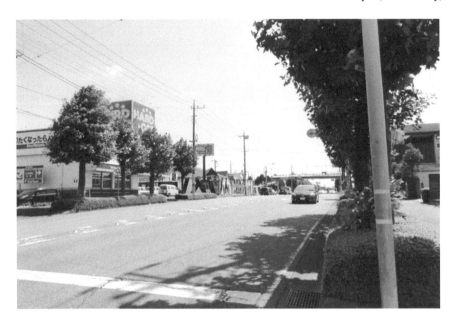

Photo 6.3 Central shopping area is located along the main streets (City D, 2015, taken by Iwama)

6.2.1   Questionnaire's Responses

We consider the living environment by the questionnaire responses. Table 6.1 shows respondents' individual attributes. Most respondents were in the 70s age group. The ratio of men to women is 47.4:52.6. This ratio is almost same as that of all age groups in this city. In terms of family structure, 86.9% of residents lived with their partners or their children, while single-person households accounted for 11.9%. Driving license rate is high in men (78.6%) and low in women (39.1%).

Table 6.2 shows their daily lives. 11.8% of the respondents feel "financial hardship". This per cent is high in women (16.1%). We analyzed "income" and "need assistance / nursing care required", but we did not find any significant differences based on living areas. 31.6% of them answered that they "stay alone during the day". The per cent of "the old person who meets with their friend and acquaintance few times per year" reached 37.3%. This tendency is remarkable in men.

The total per cent of the respondents who rarely join hobby or club activities (few times per year) was 67.5%. This per cent for men was 69.1% and women was 66.5%.[3] Figure 6.2 shows the ratio of the respondents based on each town street. This figure suggests that hobby or club activities are generally active in urban town streets, and non-active in agricultural districts.[4] However, in some urban town streets, the participation rate for hobby clubs is also low. We can see the same tendency in the participation of sports clubs. In case of neighbourhood association activities, the participation ratio is generally higher in agricultural town streets than in urban ones.

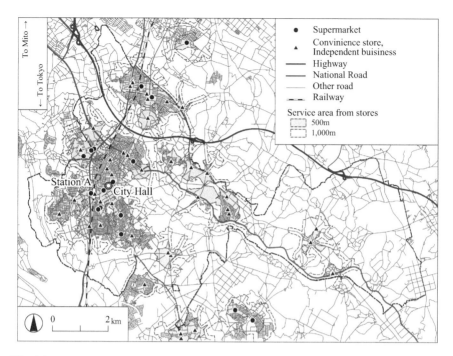

Fig. 6.1 Food access map of City D in 2015. *Source* Asakawa et al. (2016), Iwama et al. (2016)

Table 6.1   Individual attribute

(%)

Gender and age	Man	Woman	Family structure	Single	Living together with family members[a]	Other	Driving license rate	
The ratio of men to women	47.4	52.6	Total	11.9	86.9	1.1	Total	58.3
60s	31.4	29.4	Man	7.6	91.7	0.8	Man	78.6
70s	50.1	40.3	Woman	15.9	82.6	1.5	Woman	39.1
80s	16.5	23.7						
Older than 90s	2.1	6.6						
		(n = 3,984)				(n = 3,984)		(n = 3,984)

[a]Including couple household
Source Asakawa et al. (2016), Iwama et al. (2016)

Table 6.2 Elderly peoples' daily lives

(%)

Elderly people in financial hardship		Elderly people often alone during the day		Elderly people who meet friends and acquaintances several times per year		Elderly who rarely participate in hobby club activities[a]	
Total	11.8	Total	31.6	Total	37.3	Total	67.9
Men	7.1	Men	30.7	Men	43.7	Men	69.1
Women	16.1	Women	32.5	Women	31.5	Women	66.9
	(n = 2,195)		(n = 2,195)		(n = 3,984)		(n = 3,984)

[a]Amang many social activities, joining hobby clubs shows the highest correlation with the food diversity score
Source Asakawa et al. (2016), Iwama et al. (2016)

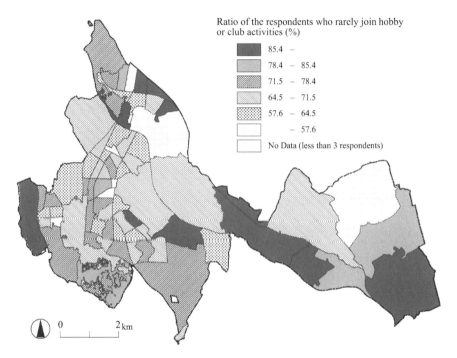

Fig. 6.2 Ratio of the respondents who rarely join hobby or club activities based on each town street in 2014. *Source* Iwama et al. (2016)

Table 6.3 suggests that high food access areas and low food access areas are mixed in City D. We calculated the average distances from the centre point of each town street to its nearest grocery stores. As a result, 13.9% of town streets have grocery stores within a 500 m radius. 41.7% of town streets have stores within a 500–1,000 m radius. On the other hand, 12.5% of town streets do not have any grocery stores within

Table 6.3 Shopping behavior

(%)

Average distance from center point of each town street to nearest grocery shop		Main mode of transport to shops	Total	Men	Women	Frequency of shopping	Total	Men	Women	Use of food delivery service		Use of mobile sales vehicle service		Elderly people who consider balance in daily diet		Elderly people who have difficulty shopping	
Within 500 m	13.9	On foot	22.9	21.6	24.0	Everyday	18.4	19.4	17.4	Total	9.8	Total	12.8	Total	59.6	Total	5.4
500–1,000 m	41.7	By bicycle	13.9	13.4	14.3	3–5 times per week	40.6	40.3	40.8	Men	8.3	Men	15.6	Men	55.9	Men	3.4
1,000–1,500 m	12.5	By bus	2.4	1.6	3.2	1–2 times per week	34.7	34.8	34.7	Women	11.1	Women	10.3	Women	63.0	Women	7.1
1,500–2,000	9.7	By taxi	0.5	0.5	0.5	1–3 times per month	4.1	3.9	4.4								
2,000–2,500	5.6	By car/motorcycle (self driven)	33.5	45.1	22.7	Others	2.2	1.7	2.8								
2,500–3,000	4.2	By car/motorcycle (driven by family members)	22.3	14.8	29.4												
over 3,000 m	12.5	Others	4.6	3.0	6.0												
(n = 72)					(n = 3,601)				(n = 3,656)		(n = 3,983)		(n = 3,983)		(n = 3,984)		(n = 3,984)

Source Asakawa et al. (2016), Iwama et al. (2016)

a 3,000 m radius. With regard to "the main transportation to go shopping", the most popular answer was "by private car" (total of 55.8%: drive by myself, 33.5% and driven by families, 22.3%). The second highest answer was "on foot" (22.9%). In general, men tend to go shopping by private cars (drive by myself), and women usually go shopping on foot or by private cars (driven by family members). With regard to the shopping frequency, more than 40% of the respondents go shopping "3-5 times per week" and only 10% go "almost every day". 9.8% of the respondents use the food delivery service. With regard to mobile selling vehicle service, 15.6% of men and 10.3% of women use this service. 59.6% of the respondents responded with "I pay attention to the nutritive balance of daily meals" (man 55.9%, women 63.0%[5]). 3.4% of men and 7.1% of women chose "I feel difficulty in daily shopping". The number of old people who are inconvenienced by daily shopping was less than expected. However, we found that the people who find it difficult to shop exist not only in poor food access agricultural areas but also in urban areas with good food access.

Table 6.4 shows the food diversity scores. The total per cent of the high-malnutrition risk in old persons (food diversity score is less than 3) was 53.5%.[6] In general, men have a higher risk of malnutrition than women. With regard to the age group, the per cent of high malnutrition risk in men is the highest in the 60s (64.2%). But those per cents decrease during the 70s (55.2%) and 80s (57.0%), and increase again in the 90s (71.7%). On the other hand, in the case of women, they retain healthy eating habits in the 60s but the per cent of high-malnutrition risk in elderly women increase during their 70s–90s.[7] The malnutrition risk per cent for the respondents who answered "I feel difficulty in daily shopping" was 67.8% and this score is relatively higher than the total average (53.5%).

Table 6.5 shows the food diversity scores of the old people based on town streets. There are 32 town streets where the ration of high-malnutrition risk elderly is more

Table 6.4 Food diversity scores (by gender and age)

	High group (%)	Low group (%)
60s men	35.8	64.2
70s men	44.8	55.2
80s men	41.1	58.9
90s men	28.9	71.1
Total (man)	41.0	59.0
60s women	55.0	45.0
70s women	54.9	45.1
80s women	43.0	57.0
90s women	37.3	62.7
Total (woman)	51.0	49.0
Total	46.5	53.5
	(n = 3,921)	

Source Asakawa et al. (2016), Iwama et al. (2016)

than 54.4% (groups A, B and C). Thirty-two town streets are about 45.1% of the total town streets in City D. The population of the old people who live in these town streets are 3,744 (45% of the total old residents). Figure 6.3 is the distribution of low-diversity scores in old residents (less than point 3). These old people mainly live in some parts of the city centre and in the fringes of the city. Fringe areas are poor food access districts. On the other hand, there are many grocery stores in the city centre and it provides high food access. However, as Fig. 6.3 suggests, the distribution of low-food diversity in old people almost corresponds to not only the low food access areas in the eastern agricultural district but also the low social capital areas in the city centre.

6.2.2   Investigation of the Factors Which Impede Old People's Healthy Eating Habits (Logistic Regression)

We now investigate the relationship between old people's healthy eating habits and their individual attributes (gender, age and income) and living environment attributes (food access and ties with families and neighbours) based on town streets. If we can find significant correlation among them, FDs exist there. In addition, this analysis might clarify which attribute strongly influences old people's healthy eating habits.

Our dataset is nested data. We calculated the average distance from houses to the nearest grocery stores based on town streets. First, we confirmed the effectiveness of multilevel analysis for this dataset. So, we checked the Intra-class Correlation Coefficient (ICC). As a result, all ICC were less than 0.1. Then, we calculated the Design Effect (DEFF) and all DEFF were less than 2. These results suggest that this dataset is not hierarchy data. Therefore, multilevel analysis is not suitable for this dataset.[8] As a result, we adopted logistic regression.[9]

Table 6.5   Food diversity scores of elderly people according to street of residence

Groups of streets (by proportion of elderly with low food-diversity scores)[a]	Number of streets[b]	%	Population > 65 years old	%
Group E: >66.1%	9	12.7	165	2.0
Group B: 60.2–66.1%	12	16.9	2,114	25.3
Group C: 54.4–60.2%	11	15.5	1,476	17.7
Group D: 48.6–54.4%	17	23.9	1,827	21.9
Group A: 42.7–48.6%	11	15.5	2,002	24.0
Group F: <42.2%	11	15.5	757	9.1

Note [a]These groups correspond to those in Fig. 6.3
[b]This list does not include some town streets that do not appear in the National Census
Source Iwama et al. (2016)

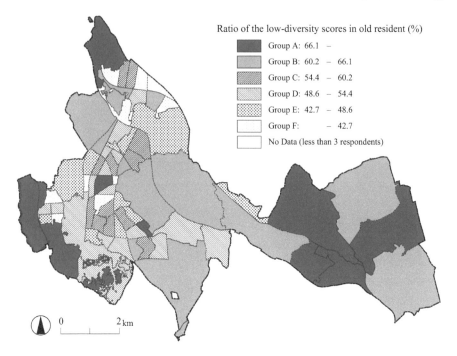

Fig. 6.3 Distribution of low-diversity scores in old residents based on each town street in 2014. *Source* Iwama et al. (2016)

6.2.2.1   Basic Attribute Model

Table 6.6 shows the result of the logistic regression. Column a shows the results of the basic attribute model. This analysis suggests the following five facts.

1.   Women have a 40% lower possibility of having a low food diversity score than men.
2.   The person in need of nursing care has 55% higher possibility of having a low food diversity score than a person who does not need nursing care.
3.   The person who has few opportunities to be alone has 15% lower possibility of having a low food diversity score than a lonely person.
4.   The person who usually dines with someone has 30% lower possibility of having a low food diversity score than a person who eats alone.
5.   The person who usually uses a car to go shopping has 20% lower possibility of having a low food diversity score than a person who does not have a private car.

Table 6.6 Logistic regression model

	a) Basic attribute		b) Basic attribute + spatial factor model		c) Basic attribute + spatial factor model + social capital		d) Mutual interaction model	
	Coefficient of regression	Odds ratio	Coefficient of regression	Odds ratio	Coefficient of regression	Odds ratio	Coefficient of regression	Odds ratio
Gender	−0.514	0.598***	−0.523	0.593***	−0.521	0.594***	−0.519	0.595***
Age	−0.011	0.989	−0.012	0.988*	−0.014	0.986*	−0.014	0.986*
Income	0.000	1.000	0.000	1.000	0.000	1.000	0.000	1.000
Family structure	0.633	1.883	0.539	1.714	0.491	1.634	0.488	1.629
Nursing care	0.437	1.548***	0.443	1.558***	0.406	1.501***	0.405	1.499***
Stay alone during the day	−0.1682	0.845**	−0.167	0.846**	−0.176	0.839**	−0.176	0.839**
Eat alone	0.234	1.264***	0.230	1.259***	0.234	1.264***	0.235	1.265***
Go shopping by car	0.169	1.184*	0.115	1.121	0.115	1.122	0.115	1.121
Distance to nearest supermarket	–	–	0.109	1.115**	0.108	1.114**	0.088	1.092
Group participation	–	–	–	–	−0.285	0.752**	−0.344	0.709**
Distance*Group participation	–	–	–	–	–	–	0.047	1.048

(continued)

Table 6.6 (continued)

	a) Basic attribute		b) Basic attribute + spatial factor model		c) Basic attribute + spatial factor model + social capital		d) Mutual interaction model	
	Coefficient of regression	Odds ratio	Coefficient of regression	Odds ratio	Coefficient of regression	Odds ratio	Coefficient of regression	Odds ratio
AIC	3266.6		3259.1		3250.3		3251.9	

Note ***$p < 0.001$, **$p < 0.01$, *$p < 0.05$

· Dependent variable: Food diversity score (0: high group, 1: low group)

· For "Gender," basic category is "men"

· For "Go shopping by car," basic category is "I do not use a car"

· For "Group participation," we use "I am a member of a hobby club" and "I am not a member of a hobby club"

The basic category is "I am not a member of a hobby club"

Source Asakawa et al. (2016)

6.2.2.2 Basic Attribute + Spatial Factor Model

Column b in Table 6.6 shows the results of the basic attribute +spatial factor model. In this analysis, "go shopping by car" was not at a significant level. So, it is clear that "go shopping by car" does not leave a significant influence on the risk of malnutrition but "distance to the nearest supermarket" leaves a significant influence on the risk of malnutrition. If the nearest grocery store is 1 km away, the risk of malnutrition will decrease by 10%.

6.2.2.3 Basic Attribute + Spatial Factor Model + Social Capital

Column c in Table 6.6 shows the results of the analysis of basic attribute + spatial factor model + social capital (the participation of hobby clubs). This table shows that the person who participates in hobby clubs' activities has a 20% lower malnutrition risk than that of a person without any club participation. Of the three models, this model shows the lowest AIC score. This model is the most suitable for our analysis.

"distance to the nearest supermarket" boosts malnutrition risk. Even after the control of this factor's effect, "group participation" still has significant effects on healthy eating habits. In addition, the interaction between "distance to the nearest supermarket" and "group participation" is not significant. So, it is safe to say that both "distance to the nearest supermarket" and "group participation" separately have significant influences to eating habits of an old person.

We also checked the influence of participating in group activities, such as volunteering, sports clubs, senior clubs, neighbourhood associations and culture schools. However, we could not find any significant relationship between food diversity scores and those group participations, except for sports clubs. Sports and health have a direct relationship. If we use "the participation of sports club" as independent variables, our analysis might be tautology. Therefore, we did not use "the participation of sports club" in our analysis.

6.2.2.4 Mutual Interaction Model

Finally, we analyzed the mutual interaction between "distance to the nearest supermarket" and "group participation". As a result, mutual interaction did not reach a significant level.

6.2.2.5 The Outline of Multi-Variable Analyses

The multi-variable analyses from above clarified the following facts.

1. Even 1 km increase in the distance between an old person's home and the nearest supermarket, increases the risk of malnutrition by 10%.

2.   The person who participates in hobby clubs has a 20% lower possibility of
     having a low-food diversity score than that of a lonely person.

6.2.3   The Verification of the FDs in City D

The above analyses suggest the existence of FDs which are caused by the deterioration
of residents' living environments. As we showed in Chapter 5, in urban areas, such
as City C, the decrease of social capital is the main cause for the urban FD issues.
On other hand, the case study of City D suggests that not only the decrease of social
capital but also the decrease of food access possibly aggravates the residents' healthy
eating habits and increases FD issues.

6.3   The Evaluations and the Tasks of Mobile Selling
Vehicle Service

6.3.1   Outline of the Service

In City D, Co-op operates the mobile selling vehicle. This service is supported by
a promotion council composed of the co-op, city hall, council of social welfare,
local elderly care management centre, incorporated non-profit organizations, and
neighbourhood associations of some town streets.[10] The vehicle's stops (the places
where the vehicle stops temporally and sells fresh foods and other items to the
neighbours) are distributed only in the areas whose neighbourhood association agrees
to provide this elderly support service.[11] There are 63 neighbourhood associations
in City D and only 24 of them had vehicle stops in 2015. The total number of vehicle
stops is 61 and 45 vehicle stops are located in City D (in September 2015).

Each vehicle stop is managed by the members of the neighbourhood association
or the welfare commissioner. They are so-called "key persons" who are trusted by the
neighbours. These key persons have a strong influence on the neighbours. These key
persons often let their neighbours (especially disadvantaged shoppers) know of the
arrival of the vehicle and suggest that they purchase their daily healthy foods there.
They, sometimes, hold food education programs in their town streets with Co-op and
invite the elderly people with poor eating habits to this program. Co-op also tries to
retain good relationships with local residents. For example, they often invite local
people to meet with them and agree to programs and communicate with them.

The base of this mobile selling vehicle service operation is the Co-op's store,
which is located in the centre of City D. The vehicle is 1.5t truck, which is improved
to be capable of carrying frozen/refrigerated foods. It is capable of carrying about
350–400 items and it goes around this city 5 days a week. Its operating time is from
10:30 to 17:00.[12] This vehicle's time table and vehicle stops are determined in detail.
The average number of vehicle stops which the vehicle makes per day is 12.2. This

vehicle stays in each vehicle stop for about 30 min. It returns to the stores at noon to restock on any shortage of fresh foods and other items. Co-op also promotes dietary education programs for the residents. This program is connected with Co-op's sales promotion. This education program is free and supported by City D's health centre. Although Co-op has tried many ways of promoting it, the total sales for this vehicle is still not profitable. This is because in the urban residential area, the main customers of this vehicle service are the wives who purchase dietary fresh ingredients at this vehicle. In agricultural areas, the main customers are elderly women who usually buy snacks and cakes there.

6.3.2   The Usage Condition of the Mobile Selling Vehicle Service

Table 6.7 shows the passenger use of this vehicle service. The average number of customer per day is 48.6, and the average total sale per day is about ¥60,000. The average expenditure per person is ¥1,237.3. On a monthly basis, the peak season is during March to May. On the other hand, the number of customers decreases in winter, summer and the rainy season (June).

Table 6.8 shows the top ten sales items. The most popular item is vegetables and its per cent of the total sales is about 12.4%. In addition, non-fresh foods, such as breads, snacks, dried noodles, ready meals (dietary dish) and lunch boxes, are also popular. Fresh meat and fresh fish are not listed in this list of top ten sales items. This fact means that many people do not use this vehicle service to retain their healthy eating habits.

Table 6.7 Passenger use of the vehicle service

	Number of customer	Total sales (10,000 yen)	Total fare per trip, per person (yen)
February	962	119	1,236
March	994	120	1,204
April[a]	1,248	151	1,211
May	1,014	127	1,253
June	934	119	1,276
July[a]	1,185	150	1,262
August	952	118	1,235
September	973	119	1,227
Total	8,262	1,022	1,237
Per day	48.6	6.0	

[a]Five weeks in April and July
Source Iwama et al. (2016)

Next, we analyze the geographical feature of this vehicle's rounding courses. Figure 6.4 shows the relation between each town street's food access and the location of the vehicle's stops.[13] Figure 6.5 shows the number of customers and total sales per

Table 6.8 Top ten sales items

Category[a]	Items sold	%
Vegetables	658	12.4
Breads and cakes	454	8.5
Snacks	449	8.4
Noodles, soybean curd, fermented soybeans, etc.	441	8.3
Fruit	434	8.2
Ready meals (dishes), and lunch boxes	292	5.5
Drinks and sweets	283	5.3
Cooked fish	259	4.9
Ice cream	240	4.5
Milk	223	4.2

[a]This category is based on Co-op
Source Iwama et al. (2016)

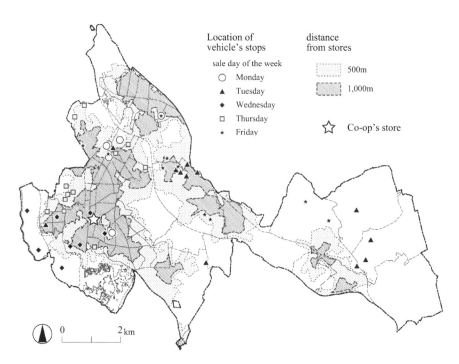

Fig. 6.4 Relation between each town street's food access and the location of the vehicle's stops in 2015. *Source* Iwama et al. (2016)

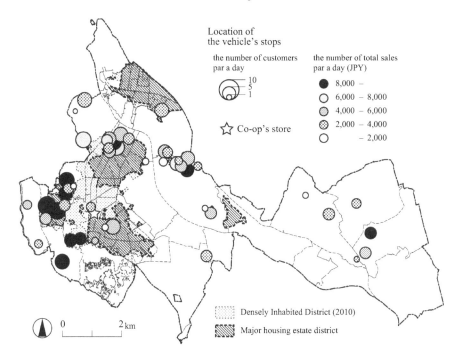

Fig. 6.5 The Number of customers and total sales par day per stop in 2015. *Source* Iwama et al. (2016)

day per stop. The location of the vehicle's stops is concentrated in the outskirts of the western high-density inhabited districts. In addition, there are also many vehicle stops within 1–2 km from the Co-op's store. On the other hand, there are few stops in the eastern poor food access areas and the city centre. The data on different days of the week show that the vehicle routes the western residential areas on Monday, Wednesday and Thursday. It goes around eastern low residential agricultural areas on Tuesday and Friday. These maps show that although this vehicle goes around some rural poor food access areas, it mainly courses the western high-density residential districts.

The number of consumers and total sales are generally high at the vehicle stops which are on the outskirts of high populated areas. Especially, these numbers of consumers and total sales are the highest in the western housing complexes. On the other hand, these numbers are lower in eastern poor food access agricultural districts.

6.3.3   The Distribution of High Malnutrition Risk in the Elderly and the Outline of the Mobile Selling Vehicle Service

6.3.3.1   The Distribution of the Mobile Selling Vehicle's Stops and the Residents' Dietary Diversity Scores

Next, we discuss the spatial relationship between the location of the vehicle stops and malnutrition risk old people's residential areas (Fig. 6.6). This figure suggests that their distribution do not correspond with each other. Table 6.9 shows the relationship between the location of the vehicle stops and each town street's ratio of malnutrition risk elderly residents. This analysis means that although some vehicle stops are established in serious poor eating habit areas, there are many exceptions. Many of the vehicle stops are established in town street cluster B (the per cent of malnutrition risk in the elderly is here more than 60.2%). The number of vehicle stops located in this cluster is 16 (30.8% of all vehicle stops). On the other hand, the number of vehicle stops which are established in cluster A (the most serious poor eating habit town street cluster; the per cent of high-malnutrition risk in the elderly here is more than 66.1%) was only 9 (17.3% of all vehicle stops). On the other hand, there are 11 vehicle stops in cluster E (the second best healthy eating habit cluster; the per

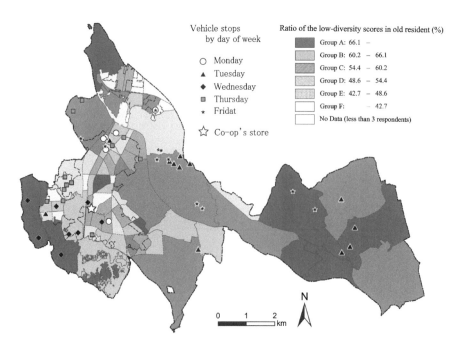

Fig. 6.6 Spatial relationship between the location of the vehicle stops and malnutrition risk old people's residential areas in 2014. *Source* Iwama et al. (2016)

Table 6.9 Relationship between location of vehicle stops and malnutrition risk of old people

Groups of streets (by proportion of elderly people with low food-diversity scores)[a]	Total		Monday	Tuesday	Wednesday	Thursday	Friday
	Number of stops	(%)	(%)	(%)	(%)	(%)	(%)
Group A: >66.1%	9	17.3	0.0	25.0	33.3	7.7	18.2
Group B: 60.2–66.1	16	30.8	33.3	58.3	0.0	15.4	45.5
Group C: 54.4–60.2	5	9.6	16.7	0.0	33.3	7.7	0.0
Group D: 48.6–54.4	7	13.5	33.3	8.3	33.3	7.7	0.0
Group E: 42.7–48.6	11	21.2	0.0	8.3	0.0	53.8	27.3
Group F: <42.2%	4	7.7	16.7	0.0	0.0	7.7	9.1

Note [a]These groups correspond to those in Fig. 6.3
Source Iwama et al. (2016)

cent of high-malnutrition risk in the elderly here is 42.7–48.6%). The vehicle goes around high malnutrition risk areas on Tuesdays and Fridays, and around healthy eating habit areas on Mondays and Thursdays.

The average malnutrition risk (the average ratio of the residents whose diversity scores are less than 3) of the town streets which have vehicle stops in their territories is 56.5%. Its standard deviation is 10.9 and the average malnutrition risk of the whole city is 55.3%. So, we could not find eating habit differences between the town areas with vehicle stops and those without any vehicle stops.

6.3.3.2 The Spatial Characteristics of the Areas Where the Elderly Need the Mobile Selling Vehicle Service

Here, we discuss the characteristics of areas where many old people need the mobile selling vehicle service from a geographical viewpoint. In particular, we investigate the special factors which contribute to the usage of this vehicle service. By this analysis, we comprehend this service's potential needs and the contribution of this service to the disadvantaged old shoppers' healthy eating habits.

First, we chose 19 variables which seemed to be related to the usage of the mobile selling vehicle service. Then, we summarized them into some six components by using the principle component analysis. Second, we conducted a multi regression analysis. The explained variable was "the usage of the vehicle services"[14] in each vehicle stop's trading areas (300 m radius areas from each vehicle stop). We used six components as explanatory variables.

As mentioned above, we chose 19 variables. As geographical variables, we chose ten variables related to residential attributes [living environments (about food access and ties with family members and neighbours)] and nine variables related to individual attributes [(about outing degree, eating habits and economic conditions)] (Table 6.10).

Table 6.10 Variables of analysis

First level	Second level	Third level	Variable
Living environment variables	Food accessibility		Accessibility of nearby grocery shops
			Drives a private car by him/herself
			Has a difficulty of shopping
	Ties with family and local community	Family	Single householder
			Stay alone in the daytime
			Number of family members
		Community	Degree of association
			Low frequency of meeting friends
			Proportion of elderly people who are not members of hobby clubs
			Proportion of people aged over 65
Variables of individual attributes	Going out		I go out more than once per week
			I can go out alone
			I can walk for more than 15 min
			I avoid going out
	Eating habits		Low score in food diversity survey
			I sometimes skip a meal
			I can prepare a meal by myself
	Economic condition		I have economic difficulties in daily life
			Low income

Source Iwama et al. (2016)

The details of the variables are as follows. First, with regard to the ten living environment variables, three variables are about food access ("food accessibility",[15] "whether they drive a private car or not" and "whether they feel difficulty in shopping"). Three variables are about the tie with family members ("single householder or not", "whether they stay alone in the daytime", "the number of family members"). Four variables are about community ("the degree of association",[16] "the frequency of meeting friends",[17] "the ratio of the old person who does not take part in hobby clubs"[18] and "the ratio of old person aged over 6 5 years"[19]).

Individual attributes are made of variables such as: four variables which are related with going out ("I go out more than once per week",[20] "I can go out alone",[21] "I can take a walk for more than 15 minutes",[22] "I refrain from going out"), three variables related to eating habits ("low score in food diversity survey", "I sometimes skip a meal",[23] "I can prepare a meal by myself"[24]) and two variables about economic conditions ("I feel difficulty in daily life economically",[25] "low income"[26]).

We extracted six main components whose characteristic value is over 1.0 (Table 6.11). The cumulative contribution of these six components is 77.6%. The primary component shows positive scores in "I go out more than once per week" and "I drive a car by myself", and negative score in "I refrain from going out". These suggest that this component is related with going out. In addition, this component also shows a positive score in "I feel difficulty in daily life economically" and a negative score in "low score in food diversity survey". This fact means that this component is also related to a healthy life. It also shows positive score in "food accessibility", and negative in "communication among neighbours" and "the number of family members". These mean the typical Characteristics of families in urban cities. Therefore, we named the primary component "urban healthy type".

The second component shows a significant positive score in "live alone" and a significant negative score in "I drive a car by myself". This component also shows positive in "I refrain from going out" and negative in "low frequency to meet friends". These are typical features of single old persons who do not drive a car and stay in their houses all day long and do not meet their friends. Therefore, we named this component "single isolated type".

The third component shows positive in "I sometime skip a meal" and negative in "I can take a walk for more than 15 minutes" and "I can go out by myself". This suggests the typical lifestyle of old people who cannot go out by themselves and sometimes skip their meals. Therefore, we named this component "bad eating habit / difficult to go out type".

The fourth component shows significant positive scores on "low income" and "I am alone in the day time" and also relatively highly positive in "I feel difficulty in daily life economically" and "low score in food diversity survey". This suggests that old residents who are alone and live in bad economic conditions, also suffer from unhealthy eating habits. So, we named this component "isolated / poverty type". Also we named the fifth component "old people type" because this component shows significant a negative score in "the rate of aging". We named the sixth component "low-sociality type" because this component shows significant positive scores in "low participation in hobby clubs" and "low frequency of meeting friends".

Table 6.11 Principal component analysis results

Variables	Primary component	Second component	Third component	Fourth component	Fifth component	Sixth component
Accessibility of nearby grocery shops	0.565*	−0.010	−0.236	−0.132	−0.178	−0.093
Drives a private car by him/herself	0.486*	−0.795**	0.154	−0.013	0.177	−0.016
Has a difficulty of shopping	0.346	0.304	0.235	−0.395	−0.483*	0.254
Single householder	0.136	0.904**	0.226	0.123	0.041	0.065
Stay alone in the daytime	−0.082	−0.050	0.172	0.766**	−0.060	−0.085
Number of family members	−0.794**	−0.053	0.444*	−0.109	0.056	−0.073
Degree of association	−0.753**	0.161	0.026	0.314	0.063	−0.325
Low frequency of meeting friends	0.246	−0.479*	0.014	−0.080	−0.183	0.674**
Proportion of elderly people are not members of hobby clubs	−0.188	0.294	0.061	−0.006	0.206	0.814**
Proportion of people aged over 65 years	−0.002	−0.021	0.096	0.196	−0.880**	−0.125
I go out more than once per week	0.789**	−0.110	0.007	−0.382	0.059	−0.065
I can go out alone	0.429*	−0.334	−0.625**	−0.340	0.118	−0.059
I can walk for more than 15 min	0.271	−0.185	−0.797**	−0.248	0.124	−0.084
I avoid going out	−0.466*	0.561*	0.346	−0.114	−0.460	0.007
Low score in food diversity survey	−0.534*	0.257	0.274	0.435*	−0.282	0.259

(continued)

Table 6.11 (continued)

Variables	Primary component	Second component	Third component	Fourth component	Fifth component	Sixth component
I sometimes skip a meal	− 0.059	− 0.034	0.903**	0.117	− 0.079	0.006
I can prepare a meal by myself	0.649**	− 0.273	− 0.101	0.156	0.379	− 0.102
I have economic difficulties in daily life	− 0.487*	− 0.171	0.115	0.539*	0.081	0.309
Low income	− 0.085	0.395	0.240	0.722**	− 0.081	− 0.065
Eigenvalue	6.408	2.376	1.908	1.572	1.361	1.124
Contribution proportion (%)	33.7	12.5	10.1	8.3	7.1	5.9
Cumulative contribution proportion (%)	33.7	46.2	56.3	64.6	71.7	77.6

* means the absolute value of factor loading is 0.4–0.6, ** means it is more than 0.6

Source Iwama et al. (2016)

Table 6.12 Results of multiple regression analysis

Explanatory variable		Partial regression coefficient	Standardized partial regression coefficient
Third component	Disability and poor eating habits	0.851	0.554***
Primary component	Urban lifestyle and interest in health	– 0.508	– 0.416***
Fourth component	Isolation and poverty	0.526	0.356**
	Constant term	1.724	***
Multiple correlation coefficient		0.766	
Coefficient of determination		0.586	
Adjusted R-square		0.571	
Goodness of model fit		$p = 0.000$	

***statistically significant at the 0.1 percent level
**statistically significant at the 1 percent level
Source Iwama et al. (2016)

Next, using these principle component scores, we carried out multi regression analysis. The explained variable is the usage of the mobile selling vehicle and explanatory variables are above principal component scores. We carried out this analysis to clarify the geographical conditions that leave a significant influence on whether the old residents of an area use this selling vehicle service or not. We did the stepwise multi regression analysis, which adopts the method of increasing and decreasing the variables. As a result, the third component, the primary component and the fourth component are adopted as the statistically significant explanatory indexes (Table 6.12).[27]

We checked the influence of these indexes by standardized partial regression coefficient scores. The third component shows the highest influence (positive). The primary component shows the second highest influence (negative) and it is followed by the fourth component (positive).

These results suggest the following points. ① The more the number of elderly residents with problems of disability and poor eating habits increase, the more the usage of the vehicle service increases (the third component). ② The more the number of old residents with an urban lifestyle and interest in health increase, the more the usage of the vehicle service in the area decrease (the primary component). ③ The more the number of old residents with isolation and poverty increase, the more the usage of the vehicle service in the area increase (fourth component).

So, it is safe to say that there is high potential demand in these areas where there are many old residents with the problems of disability, isolation from neighbours and poverty (= urban FDs). On the other hand, there seems to be few demands in the areas where residents live in an urban style and care for healthy eating habits.

6.3.4 The Evaluation to the Mobile Selling Vehicle Service in City D

The above analyses point out the following five facts. (1) In City D, the grocery stores are located mainly in the western urban areas and there are large poor food access areas in the eastern agricultural districts. However, many residents use their private cars and generally do not feel difficulty in shopping daily. (2) The per cent of high-malnutrition risk in an old person is 53.5%. These high-risk old people mainly live in urban city centres (high food access areas) and agricultural districts (poor food access areas). (3) Many vehicle stops are established in the housing complexes located in the outskirts of the city centre. Food access in these housing complexes is relatively high. There is a gap between the location of the vehicle stops and high-malnutrition risk elderly people's residential areas. (4) The usage of mobile selling vehicle service is high in the areas where many old people with problems of disability and poor eating habits live and in the areas where many old people are isolated from society and suffer from poverty. On the other hand, the usage of this service is low in the areas where residents live in an urban lifestyle and have healthy eating habits.

There is no doubt that the mobile selling vehicle service in City D contributes to the improvement of the living environment of disadvantaged shoppers. This service also plays an important role in supporting the elderly with disability, isolation and poverty issues. Therefore, we evaluate this service highly in these points.

On the other hand, we found some problems. First is the location of the vehicle stops. The locations of the vehicle stops have not fully covered the area of high-malnutrition risk elderly people's residences. There seems to be many old people who really need the shopping support services. This vehicle service might improve the poor eating elderly's dietary habits. So, we should clarify the distribution of high-malnutrition risk elderly people's residences exactly and establish the vehicle stops there.

Second is a cooperation between the mobile shopping vehicle service and dietary education programs. From this survey, we clarified that many residents in City D thought that they maintained healthy eating habits. However, in fact, more than half of them were suffering from high-malnutrition risk. This fact means that many residents are blind to their unhealthy eating habits. The list of foods which residents purchase at the mobile selling vehicle mainly consists of non-fresh foods, such as breads and snacks. To improve residents' eating habits, we should pay attention not only to the improvement of food access but also to fresh and healthy foods' purchase promotion. This promotion must be corroborated by food retailers (mobile selling vehicle) and the public health insurance centre (dietary education).

Actually, there are many restrictions and difficulties in the mobile selling vehicle service. To suppress delivery costs, the vehicle has to refrain from going around remote and low-density populated areas. Even if the usage ratio of the residents is high, the total number of customers in remote and rural areas is much lower than those of urban areas. It is inefficient to establish many vehicle stops in remote and rural areas. In the first place, it is impossible to establish vehicle stops in town streets where the neighbourhood associations do not accept this disadvantaged shoppers' supporting services. It is mainly because of these restrictions that the service blank areas exist widely in City D. Also, in the case of residents who do not have any interest in healthy eating, no matter how much and how many kinds of fresh foods the vehicle carries, the residents might not purchase them.

In addition, there is another big restriction when we try to locate the residences of old people who need shopping support services. The users of the mobile selling vehicle service have changed rapidly in a short period of time. The main users of this service are old people who support themselves enough to cook, but hardly go shopping to a distant grocery store by themselves. However, if their self-support degree decreases, they need careful welfare supports. On the other hand, it becomes difficult with age to go shopping. So, the number of old people who need shopping support is continuously increasing. It is very difficult for retailers to keep collecting information of the old people with shopping disadvantages by their own efforts.

We must maintain, at least, an essential shopping environment in remote and rural areas. However, almost all shopping support services in these areas are operated in debt. Many of them are operated by private companies or non-profit organisations (NPOs). The government should provide essential shopping support services in these areas and support these services economically from a social welfare viewpoint.[28] To promote dietary education support, collaboration between the retailers and the public health care centres is necessary. In addition, for clarifying the location of elderly people in need of support, cooperation between retailers, the government, residents and researchers is necessary. The local government has detailed information about old residents' personal data, including individual attributes, their economic condition, medical condition, etc. But the disclosure of these personal data is severely restricted and, sometimes, this huge amount of information is not organized. Unorganized information is quite inconvenient for researchers to analyze. If these huge amount of data is compiled into a database and shared with researchers from various fields (after the database is adapted for the protection of personal information), useful analyses can be conducted, such as knowing the exact location of elderly people in need of support (who exactly needs this support), provision of needs (what kinds of support do these old people really need) and future simulation (who will need this support in the near future and what kind of support will they need in the near future). These analyses will make the elderly supporting services more effective and sustainable.

It is difficult for the government to back specific commercial companies, such as Co-op. So, some cities have decided against supporting all mobile selling vehicle services due to their position as an evenhanded government. However, in many cases, including City D, many retailers who manage mobile selling services bear the deficit expense by themselves from a social welfare viewpoint. Actually, these disadvantaged shopper supporting services are a kind of social welfare activity. FD issues will become more serious in the near future. We have to establish sustainable and effective elderly support systems. To realize these systems, the cooperation between the government, retailers, residents and researchers is essential.

6.4 The Outline of This Chapter

In this chapter, we discussed the existence of FDs and analyzed the significant living environment factors that trigger FD issues. In this research, we did a large scale questionnaire surveys and statistical analyses. The case study city was a small city, D, which has different types of areas: urban residential areas for commuters going to Tokyo and the agricultural areas where many farmers have lived for many generations. In addition, we assessed the mobile selling vehicle service operating in the city. We found that shopping destination blank areas are largely located in the eastern agricultural areas of this city. However, high malnutrition risk old people live not only in these poor food access agricultural areas but also in the city centres which maintains good food access. Our surveys suggest that there are two main living environmental factors which exacerbate old residents' healthy eating habits: local level social capital (a weak tie with family members and neighbours) and food access (poor shopping environment). Social capital significantly influences elderly people's healthy eating habits in urban areas and food access significantly influences the same in agricultural areas.

The mobile selling vehicle supports disadvantaged old residents' daily lives. For some old residents, this service is their lifeline. However, the vehicle stops are mainly established around housing complexes and do not fully cover high malnutrition risk elderly people's residential areas, such as poor food access areas in eastern agricultural areas and the weak social capital areas in the western city centre. Our analyses suggest that the usage of the mobile selling vehicle is high not only in the areas where there are many old people with difficulty in going out on foot (low food access areas), but also in the areas where there are many elderly who suffer from isolation and poverty (poverty areas and low social capital areas). We should consider shopping support service again from the viewpoint of FD issues and improve this problem.

Notes

1. This data is based on the income level list by public long-term care insurance. This insurance classifies the elderly into eight groups according to their economic condition.
2. In this chapter, we measured the elderly person's tie with families and neighbours using these two indexes: the participation of vertical and horizontal organizations (neighbourhood associations and local clubs, such as sports clubs and hobby clubs), and the frequency of communicating with their neighbours (the existence of a person to dine together with, the frequency of dining together). There are two types of social capital: structural social capital and recognition social capital. The above indexes are categorized as structural social capital. These indexes are widely used by governments and in many academic fields. Structural social capital is suitable for our research. Therefore, we have not used recognition social capital in our research.

3.   Among hobby clubs, sports clubs and neighbourhood associations, hobby clubs showed the highest participation rate. Recently, the participation rate of neighbourhood associations is decreasing throughout the nation (Ministry of Economy, Trade and Industry, 2014). Hobby club activities (lifetime educations) are good occasions for the residents to promote cultural exchange with neighbours and to revitalize the local community (Ministry of Land, Infrastructure, Transport, 2005).

4.   In agricultural areas, the persons who often participate in hobby clubs and sports clubs are evaluated negatively because rural people consider these people to be lazy.

5.   We asked the following question to the residents. "What do you regard the most important in a daily diet? Please choose the most suitable answer from alternatives (up to 2). ① I eat what I want to eat. ② Do not eat too much. I eat what I want to eat. ③ Something easy to eat and drink. ④ Price (cheaper price). ⑤ Nutrition balance. ⑥ Something easy to cook. ⑦ Nothing special. The ratio means the per cent of the elderly who choose.

6.   We analyzed the FD issues using the same research method. This score (53.5%) is similar with those of other cities.

7.   Generally, the following facts are widely known. ① Compared with women, men fall into bad eating habits easily. ② Generally, the aging generation prefers a healthy diet.

8.   Multilevel analysis is suitable for hierarchical data which is nested structure. For details, please see Chapter 8, note 8.

9.   This is a kind of multiple regression analysis. This analysis quantitatively clarifies the relationship between one result (explained variable) and some factors which seem to specifically influence explained variables (explanatory variables). This analysis is popular in epidemiology and sociological researches.

10. The council assists this mobile selling vehicle service. Our researches possibly contribute to support their service and might solve the FD issues in this city. Therefore, the council fully supported our researches in city D.

11. Some neighborhood associations have prejudices, such as "all of our neighbours have private cars. We also often help each other. So, we are sure that there must be no disadvantaged shoppers in our town street". These perceptions cause people to reject this mobile selling vehicle service. In general, these reactions are common in agricultural areas. However, there are many old residents isolated and without a car there. On the other hand, in case of urban areas, there are many residents who are not so positive to neighborhood association activities. They do not like to increase their burdens and reject supporting the mobile selling vehicle service.

12. They load fresh foods and other items from their supermarket. The store opens at 10:00 a.m. So, they load foods and other goods from 10:00 to 10:30. The vehicle starts operating at around 10:30.

13. There are 48 vehicle stops in City D. 36% of these stops are located at the front of private houses.

14. We calculated "usage of the vehicle services" by the following formula. "usage of the vehicle services" = "the total number of customers" ÷ "trade area population" "trade area population" is 300 m radius area from each vehicle stop. We estimated "trade area population" using residential polygons of a housing map (published by ZENRIN CO., LTD.).

15. We measured "store accessibility" by the following formula. Equation (6.1) is a gravity model potential accessibility (Tanaka 2004). In this model, we substituted polygon area by ZMapTownII (published by ZENRIN CO., LTD.) for store size.

$$A_i = \sum_{k=1}^{n} \left(\frac{S_j}{d_{ij}^2} \right) \tag{6.1}$$

A_i means store accessibility at vehicle stop i, S_j means the polygon area of store j, and d_{ij} means the shortest road distance between vehicle stop i and store j.

16. We asked the residents about the relationship with their neighbours. This index means the per cent of the residents who answered "we often consult and help each other".

17. We asked the residents about the frequency of meeting with their friends and acquaintances. This index means the per cent of the residents who answered "a few times per year or more less."

18. We asked the residents about their frequency of participating in hobby clubs. This index means the per cent of the residents who answered "a few times per year or more less."

19. Based on the National Census, 2010.

20. We asked the residents "do you go out more than once per week?". This index means the per cent of residents who answered "yes".

21. We asked the residents "can you go outside by yourself?". This index means the per cent of residents who answered "yes". This is the index to determine their degree of self-support.

22. We asked the residents "can you take a work for more than 15 minutes?". This index means the per cent of old people who answered "yes".

23. We asked the residents "do you sometimes skip your meal?". This index means the per cent of residents who answered "yes, everyday" or "yes, few times per week".

24. We asked the residents "can you prepare your meal by yourself?". This index means the per cent of residents who answered "yes I can and actually I do" or "yes I can but now I do not prepare by myself".

25. We asked the residents "how do you think of your life from an economical viewpoint?". This index means the per cent of residents who answered "I feel difficulty".

26. This ratio means the per cent of the three lower income groups of public long-term care insurance system.

27.   *P*-value was 0.05.
28.   For example, in Kohu town, Tottori prefecture, the town government outsources the safety confirmation work for the elderly to the mobile selling vehicle company. The government offers the subsidies to this company. This company makes up for the deficit of the vehicle service by these subsidies and maintains the shopping support services. Recently, some city governments emulated this case study and supported their local mobile selling vehicle company economically.

References

Asakawa T, Iwama N, Tanaka K, Komaki N (2016) Food desert issues in a local city: empirical study in a local city that is composed of urban and rural area. Ann Jpn Assoc Urban Sociol 34:93–106 (Japanese)

Iwama N, Tanaka K, Komaki N, Ikeda M, Asakawa T (2016) Mapping residential areas of elderly people at high risk of undernutrition: analysis of mobile sales vehicles from the viewpoint of food desert issues. J Geogr 125(4):583–606 (Japanese)

Tanaka K (2004) Trends and issues in accessibility studies in the GIS era. Geog Rev Jpn 77(14):977–996 (Japanese)

Part II
FD Risk in the Affected Areas of the Great East Japan Earthquake

This book mainly introduces Japanese urban Food Desert (FD) issues. In general, urban space structures, including the distribution of population and industries, are changing constantly in all cities. When urban structures change, 'distortions', called 'spatial hole' and 'social hole' in Chap. 1, must occur in some areas of the cities. FD issue is a serious problem for the people who fall into these 'distortions' (IWAMA et al. 2011). These spatial and social holes are generally formed across a few decades. However, in the case of disaster-struck areas, these holes are formed suddenly and dramatically.

The Great East Japan Earthquake occurred on 11th May 2011. Eight years have passed since this dreadful disaster. Even now, many local people suffer from many difficulties. The number of refugees from this disaster is still at about 5,400 in January 2019 (Japanese Reconstruction Agency). Our research team has researched one of the disaster areas—Yamada town from the Iwate prefecture—from June 2011 up to the present. We met many local people and conducted interview surveys about their living environments. We also interviewed the local government and commerce and industrial companies, and we analysed the restoration and reconstruction status of social infrastructures, including shopping environments. Many people have tried hard to reconstruct these disaster areas. We commend their efforts.

Through these researches, it is clear that spatial and social holes are emerging after the disaster (Table 1). Yamada is a typical fishing town. Before the earthquake, many residents of Yamada went shopping at suburban supermarkets. The central shopping streets of this town were mostly shut at that time, although there were some small independent stores in each settlement of this town and these family-run stores supported local villagers' daily lives. In addition, this town depended on marine products and social ties among residents were very strong. Their living environments changed suddenly after the earthquake. Many settlements located in seaside areas were seriously damaged by the tsunami and big fire. Almost 80% of the houses and stores were destroyed, and surviving residents escaped to evacuation shelters. Due to the natural disaster, many shelters suffered from serious food shortages.

It was only after one month that foods and commodity goods were distributed to disaster areas by Japan' s Self-Defense Forces, the government, and many volunteers

Table 1 Living environment of Yamada Town

		Spacial viewpoint	Social viewpoint	Background of Food desert issues
Before the disaster		Many residents used suburban supermarkets, but individual stores also operated in each district.	Yamada is a typical fishing town, and residents had strong ties with the local community.	There were relatively large 'spatial hole' (poor food access areas). However, 'strong social ties' made up for their inconvenient living environments.
After the disaster	Evacuation shelters	Almost all grocery stores disappeared. However, food and commodities were distributed to shelters by the Self-Defense Forces, the government and many volunteers.	Residents escaped to nearby shelters. Therefore, each shelter was occupied by local people from the same district. Displaced persons retained strong ties with their neighbors.	Spatial holes' are becoming much larger. However, 'strong social ties' still make up for their living environments.
	Temporary houses	Many stores opened in Yamada Town. However, people in some temporary houses in remote districts suffered from poor food access.	People chose temporary houses according to their wishes. Therefore, local communities were broken up. Displaced persons had to build new social ties with new neighbors.	Large 'spatial holes' and 'social holes' are emerging. Food desert issues might occur (or many have already occured) in the disaster areas.

Source Interview survey

from all over the world. Thanks to them, shelters' food shortage was reduced. At the same time, a few local retailers restarted their businesses by restocking from their stone warehouses, which had escaped the tsunami and the flames. Also, some local retailers restarted their businesses at temporary stores. In addition, a few retailers started mobile selling vehicle services (Photos 1–2). Because the local residents had escaped into evacuation shelters with their neighbours, they could maintain their intimate local level social capital and help each other in the shelters. Fortunately, some houses on hills escaped the tsunami and the fire. But it is said that the families from these houses found it difficult to stay at evacuation shelters, because people who lost their family members and houses were envious of these relatively less-affected people.

Yamada's basic infrastructure (i.e., recovery of water pipes and electric lines, removal of debris from roads, etc.) had almost recovered three months after the earthquake. At that time, the temporary population of this town rapidly increased because many volunteers who engaged in refugees' care and construction workers who engaged in reconstruction work came to Yamada. Then, some retail chains started opening new convenience stores, supermarkets, and do-it yourself stores in suburban areas of this town (Figure 1, Photo 3). Opening these new stores developed Yamada's shopping environments. On the other hand, these changes led to concerns over the serious possibility that many old people without cars would fall into the category of disadvantaged shoppers. Earlier, individual stores had offered foods and commodity goods to old people with poor food access who lived in rural areas far from the town centre. These stores had also been important places for the elderly to congregate at for communicating and exchanging information with each other. However, many of these individual stores closed at this time (within three months of the earthquake) (Photo 4).

Photo 1 Temporary store using warehouse, (Yamada Town, 2011, taken by Iwama)

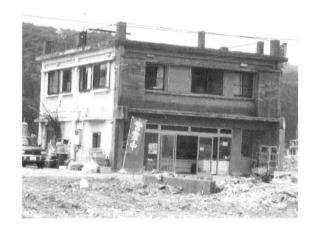

Photo 2 Mobile vending vehicle in temporary houses (Yamada Town, 2011, taken by Komaki)

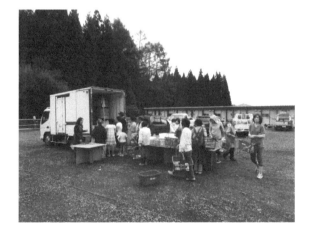

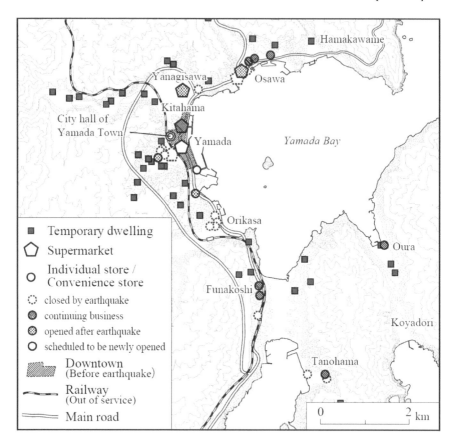

Figure 1   Location of grocery stores in Yamada Town (2017)

Photo 3   Suburban
supermarket (Yamada Town,
2011, taken by Komaki)

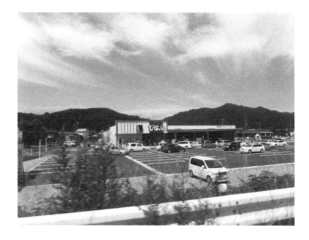

Photo 4 Urban
redevelopment project in
central area of Yamada Town
and closed temporary stores.
(Yamada Town, 2015, taken
by Komaki)

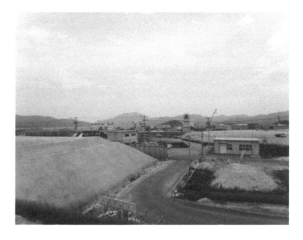

    With regard to social capital, thanks to the local council of social welfare's
and many volunteers' efforts, many people's social ties with their neighbours had
been reconstructed at evacuation shelters and temporary housing estates. However,
recently, these ties are becoming weaker. It is because many people, especially the
young and wealthy, rebuild their livelihoods and leave from the temporary housing
estates to their new houses. In many cases, these people were key persons at the
temporary housing estates' communities. Now, many poor/old people still live in
temporary housing estates and suffer from a higher risk of isolation from society.

    As I mentioned above, FD in The Great East Japan Earthquake's disaster areas are
basically based on 'distortions' which were formed by the earthquake and fire. The
speed of enlarging FDs in these areas is much faster than those of standard FDs (i.e.,
FDs in remote areas and inner areas of big cities). Recently, the Japanese government
and researchers have begun to once again pay attention to urban development with
the view of pre-disaster improvement planning. We should consider how to make
efficient safety nets against social and special holes in disaster areas.

    Eight years have passed since we started FD research in the town of Yamada.
Local people still suffer from the aftereffects of the earthquake. It would be our
great pleasure if our research can, in any way, contribute to the development of these
disaster areas.

References

Iwama N (ed) (2011) Food desert issues: food deserts and isolated society. Association of Agriculture
    and Forestry Statistics, Tokyo (Japanese)
Iwama N, Sasaki M, Tanaka K, Komaki N, and Asakawa T (2013) Recovery process of the
    food distribution system in a disaster-affected area and living conditions of disaster victims
    in temporary housing. E journal GEO 7(2):178–196 (Japanese with English abstract)

Chapter 7
Measures to Address Food Desert Issues

Abstract The purposes of this chapter are to classify the services and management measures to address Food Desert (FD) issues in Japan and to introduce some striking examples. Counter-measures against shopping disadvantage can be classified into three types: 'Dining together', 'Food deliveries', and 'Improving food access'. It is impossible to sustain unprofitable businesses, even when they are useful for disadvantaged shoppers. Not only questions such as 'what kinds of services should we provide?' but also 'how should we provide services?' are important. Some have noted this point and created new businesses. We have classified these new counter-measures into seven types: "Business Expansion", "Entry from a Different Industry", "Co-operation with Different Industries", "Resident Volunteering", "Co-operation with Industry", "Government, Scholars, and the Local Community", "Welfare businesses", and "New Businesses". We discuss the details of each type of service.

Keywords Measures to address food desert issues · Classification by service contents · Classification by management · Volunteer taxi passenger transportation by private vehicle

7.1 Support Services for Disadvantaged Shoppers

The purposes of this chapter are to classify the services and management measures to address Food Desert (FD) issues in Japan and to introduce some striking examples. Eight years have passed since the Japanese government implemented many support services for disadvantaged shoppers (providing subsidies to private companies and non-profit organizations that operate such services). During this period, many services were planned and implemented. Some operators continue to provide their services, but many others could not sustain their services and have discontinued them.

7.1.1 The Classification of Support Services for Disadvantaged Shoppers (FD Measures)

In our previous book in 2010, we classified counter-measures against shopping disadvantage into three types: 'Dining together', 'Food deliveries', and 'Improving food access'. Then we discussed the characteristics of each service from the viewpoints of sustainability, profitability, and versatility (Iwama 2011) (Table 7.1). Dining together refers to a kind of dining party with neighbours. The purpose of such parties is to create outside activities for isolated elderly people who usually stay in their houses and seldom go out. Outside activities are a form of preventative care. In addition, these dining parties are expected to be good opportunities for the elderly to make friends and participate in society. This may also protect isolated elderly people from so-called 'dying alone' issues. These parties are usually held several times per month.

Food deliveries include food deliveries, meal deliveries, and shopping services (shopping on behalf of an elderly person). These services are mainly provided to those with physical disabilities, disadvantaged shoppers, and single elderly people (including those with a family but who usually stay alone at home during the day).

Improving food access includes opening new shops and operating mobile vending vehicle services and shopping buses. These types of support are usually offered to people living in poor food access areas without private cars or access to public transportation. These three classifications of FD counter-measures correspond to those laid down by the Japanese Ministry of Economy, Trade and Industry in 2010 (Ministry of Economy, Trade and Industry 2019).

Table 7.2 shows the major measures of poor food access as of 2016. There are still three types of counter-measures: dining together, food deliveries, and improving food access. However, a few new trials have been undertaken since 2010. For example, mobile vending vehicles sell commodities in agricultural villages, purchasing fresh local foods in those areas and selling them in other villages and towns. Some local governments collaborate with researchers like us to clarify the FD issues and find out more about the health of elderly residents (quantitative research on the distribution of elderly people whose eating habits have been deteriorated by FDs and the kinds of support required). Deregulation of volunteer taxi passenger transportation by private vehicles is also an important change (NPO Zenkoku-ido Service Network 2015) (for more detail, see Sect. 7.2.7).

Table 7.1 Countermeasures against shopping disadvantage

Type of service	Dining together	Food delivery	Improving food access
Countermeasures	Dinner parties with neighbors	Food deliveries, meal deliveries, shopping for an elderly person	Opening new shops, mobile vending vehicle, shopping bus

Source Iwama ed. (2011)

Table 7.2 List of disadvantaged shopper support services (countermeasures against food desert issues) in Japan in 2020

	Countermeasure	Operating body (name)	Operating body	Partner	Area of operation	Year of establishment	Outline of services	Classification by management	Source
• Dining together • Improving food access	• Dining together, • Meal delivery	NPO corporations: Sasae Au Kai Minori	• NPO (nonprofit organization)		Inagi City, Tokyo Pref.	1984	This NPO offers many elderly welfare services including dinner parties, a meal delivery service, a day care service, and other services commissioned by local government	• Resident volunteering	(1) Our own research
	• Opening new shop • Dining together	NPO corporations: Kurashi Kyodokan Nakayoshi	• NPO		Hitachinaka City, Ibaraki Pref.	2006	Nalayoshi has repurposed a closed cooperative shop to open its own shop where it offers a wide range of fresh foods, a restaurant, a café, and other facilities to local residents. This NPO also manages some culture clubs. This shop is staffed by volunteers (Sect. 7.2.3)	• Resident volunteering	Our own research

(continued)

Table 7.2 (continued)

Countermeasure	Operating body (name)	Operating body	Partner	Area of operation	Year of establishment	Outline of services	Classification by management	Source
• Creation of elderly people's sustainable community space • Free bus • Welfare non-free transportation	• Fukushi Life • Icora Mall Izumisano • Tokyo Rope MFG Co., Ltd • Fureai center & Salon	• A general incorporated association • Shopping centre • Developer • Volunteer group		Izumisano City, Osaka Pref.	2017	This is a new type of business to support the elderly by creating sustainable and free community spaces with convenient transport. The unique aspects of this business are (1) The S.C. pays almost all the expenses of this community space and provides a free bus, and (2) it offers a paid welfare transport service for elderly people who need care or support (Sect. 7.2.7)	• New businesses	Our own research

(continued)

Table 7.2 (continued)

	Countermeasure	Operating body (name)	Operating body	Partner	Area of operation	Year of establishment	Outline of services	Classification by management	Source
• Delivery	• Meal delivery	Seven-Eleven Japan (Seven meal service)	• Convenience store		• Whole country	2012	Seven-Eleven has developed many kinds of home-delivered meals that are well balanced and easy to cook. This company operates a home-delivery service on a nationwide scale using its logistic systems and shop networks	• Business expansion	(2)
	• Food delivery	Coconet	• Logistic company	• Supermarket	• South Ward and Jonan Ward, Hukuoka City, Fukuoka Pref. • Some other big cities	2012	Coconet is affiliated with a local supermarket. This company receives orders from supermarket customers by phone, fax, internet, etc., and delivers orders to their customers' houses by the next day at the latest	• Entry from a different industry • Cooperation with different industries	(1)

(continued)

Table 7.2 (continued)

Countermeasure	Operating body (name)	Operating body	Partner	Area of operation	Year of establishment	Outline of services	Classification by management	Source
• Food delivery	Yamoto Transport	• Logistic company	• Municipality • Society of Commerce and Industry	• Whole country	2012	Yamoto is one of the largest logistic companies in Japan. This company has developed support services for disadvantaged shoppers throughout the country. It is affiliated with many local shopping streets and operates home delivery services for customers of local shops. Local governments and local chambers of commerce support Yamoto to lighten the burden of this service	• Entry from a different industry • Cooperation with different industries	(3)
• Food delivery	• Fuji Supermarket • Japan Post network	• Supermarket	• Post office	Yahatanishi Ward, Kitakyushu City, Fukuoka Pref.	2012	This supermarket has a system for orders and the catalogue. This shop commissions local post offices to collect order sheets and deliver goods to customers	• Entry from a different industry • Cooperation with different Industries	(1)

(continued)

Table 7.2 (continued)

Countermeasure	Operating body (name)	Operating body	Partner	Area of operation	Year of establishment	Outline of services	Classification by management	Source
• Manufacture and delivery of meals	Family Network Systems (Onemile)	• Meal manufacture company	• Wholesale sake merchants	15 prefectures	1988	This company manufactures original frozen meals that are cooked based on advice from specialists including chefs, nutritionists, and medical doctors, so they taste good, are of quality and nutritionally balanced. The company sells these meals using a regular customer visiting system. This company was originally a wholesaler of sake (Japanese rice wine) and it has a wide network of liquor shops. By using this network and its distribution system, the company reduces the delivery costs of frozen meals	• New businesses • Cooperation with different industries	(1) Our own research

(continued)

Table 7.2 (continued)

	Countermeasure	Operating body (name)	Operating body	Partner	Area of operation	Year of establishment	Outline of services	Classification by management	Source
• Delivery • Improving food access	• Mobile vending vehicle • Food delivery	Sanwa limited company	• Convenience store (third party)	• Municipality • Local company • Self-community Association	• Shinsaka District and Kusaki District, Jinsekikougen Town, Hiroshima Pref.	2012	This mobile vending vehicle service is based in a convenience store. These districts are true poor food access areas and the convenience store is managed by a third party. A local company employs a manager for this vehicle (sales and delivery). Local residents and neighborhood associations support the vehicle service. The vehicle also provides a service by watching elderly people and receives subsidies from the local government	• Cooperation with different industries	(1)

(continued)

Table 7.2 (continued)

Countermeasure	Operating body (name)	Operating body	Partner	Area of operation	Year of establishment	Outline of services	Classification by management	Source
• Improving food access								
• Mobile vending vehicle	Adachi Shoji (Aikyo)	• Mobile vending vehicle • Supermarket	• Municipalities	Hino Town and Kofu Town, Tottori Pref.	1990	Adachi shoji is the pioneer mobile vending vehicle company in Japan. However, owing to a rapid decrease in the local population, the management of this service has deteriorated recently. However, with a deep knowledge of all communities in its business area, this company complements the welfare function of the local government. As a result, the company offsets losses from its retail business. (Sect. 7.2.4)	• Welfare businesses	Our own research
• Volunteer taxi passenger transportation	NPO corporations: Fukushi life	• NPO		• Whole country	2006	This NPO provides open lectures all over the country to train drivers for no-fee welfare transportation	• New businesses	Our own research

(continued)

Table 7.2 (continued)

Countermeasure	Operating body (name)	Operating body	Partner	Area of operation	Year of establishment	Outline of services	Classification by management	Source
• Mobile vending vehicle	• Palette supermarket • Asuke Commerce and Industry Association	• Supermarket • Shopping Street Promotion Association	• Supermarket • Shopping Street Promotion Association	Toyota City, Iichi Pref.	2012	These companies operate two mobile vending vehicles. One is operated by a supermarket and sells many kinds of food. The other is provided by the Commerce and Industry Association of this city and mainly sells commodity goods	• Business expansion • Cooperation with different industries	(1)
• Mobile vending vehicle	Social welfare authority: Kagyu Sankei Kai	• Social welfare corporation	• Shopping Street Promotion Association	Kakuta City, Miyaghi Pref.	2011	This vehicle is operated by the social welfare corporation and it offers many foods in poor food access areas. This vehicle sells bread and meals cooked by their facilities' occupants. This vehicle also purchases many goods from individual neighborhood shops at a discount (20% off) and sells them in poor food access area	• Cooperation with different industries	(1)

(continued)

Table 7.2 (continued)

Countermeasure	Operating body (name)	Operating body	Partner	Area of operation	Year of establishment	Outline of services	Classification by management	Source
• Opening new shops	JA (Japan Agricultural Cooperatives) Yutaka	• Farmers' cooperative	• Yamazaki baking (Breadmaking company)	Kure City, Hiroshima Pref.		JA's small shop was in a management crisis because of the decreasing population and aging of residents. Therefore, the shop joined the Yamazaki baking group (The largest Japanese breadmaking company. This company has nationwide food distribution systems). Using Yamazaki's distribution systems and group buying networks, the JA shop cut its running costs and also improved the quality of service to customers	• Cooperation with different industries	(2)

(continued)

Table 7.2 (continued)

Countermeasure	Operating body (name)	Operating body	Partner	Area of operation	Year of establishment	Outline of services	Classification by management	Source
• Volunteer taxi passenger transportation	NPO corporations: Nakasato	• NPO	• Municipality	Hitachi City, Ibaraki Pref.	2009	Local people established an NPO to operate a volunteer taxi passenger service (they have two on-demand buses). This NPO raises funds for the vehicles' running costs through taxi fees, membership fees from all residents, and subsidies from local government	• Cooperation with different industries	Our own research

(continued)

Table 7.2 (continued)

Countermeasure	Operating body (name)	Operating body	Partner	Area of operation	Year of establishment	Outline of services	Classification by management	Source
• Volunteer taxi passenger transportation	Sai Village Social Welfare Council	• Social welfare councils	• Municipality • Local residents • Supermarket	Sai Village, Aomori Pref.	2005	The local social welfare council operates a volunteer taxi passenger transportation service. Many local people with driving licenses have registered as volunteer drivers. The council is in charge of matching jobs (receiving orders from customers and allocating on-demand buses). When a registered driver take customers (car-less old residents) to a local supermarket by an on-demand car, drivers receive stamps from the supermarket. The driver can exchange these stamps for supermarket coupons	• Cooperation with different industries • Resident volunteering	(2)

(continued)

Table 7.2 (continued)

Countermeasure	Operating body (name)	Operating body	Partner	Area of operation	Year of establishment	Outline of services	Classification by management	Source
• Mobile vending vehicle	Ibaraki Co-op	• Cooperative society	• Municipality • Researchers	Mito City and Ushiku City, Ibaraki Pref.	2011	This wagon is operated by promotion committee consisting of a cooperative, the local government, local people, and an NPO. The promotion committee cooperated with researchers and clarified the food desert issues in the city. It shares the database for this research and uses this information to develop their wagon operations. (Sect. 7.2.1)	• Government, scholars, and the local community	Our own research

(continued)

Table 7.2 (continued)

Countermeasure	Operating body (name)	Operating body	Partner	Area of operation	Year of establishment	Outline of services	Classification by management	Source
• Mobile vending vehicle	Tokushimaru	• Mobile vending vehicle business management company	• Supermarket • Local company	• Whole country	2012	This company established a nationwide franchise system of mobile vending vehicle business. Supermarkets and wagon drivers become franchisees of this company. Drivers have single-proprietorships. Drivers purchase fresh food from local supermarkets and sell them in their living areas	• Cooperation with different industries • Business expansion	Our own research

(continued)

Table 7.2 (continued)

Countermeasure	Operating body (name)	Operating body	Partner	Area of operation	Year of establishment	Outline of services	Classification by management	Source
• Shopping bus	Hokuto City local public transportation revitalization council	• Local residents	• Local residents • Researchers	Hokuto City, Yamenashi Pref.	2009	A council (cooperative) is in charge of making plans, operating a vehicle service and bears the financial burdens. Local people give exact information about their needs for a shopping support service. The researchers have introduced a new management system of an on-demand bus to the council and support its smooth operations	• Government, scholars, and the local community • Resident volunteering	(2)
• Opening new shops	NPO corporations: Yabakei Noson Club	• NPO	• Local residents • Supermarket	Nakatsu City, Oita Pref.	2005	Residents of a poor food access area established a NPO and opened the shared cooperative shop. They also started commissioned sales of local agricultural products at supermarkets to earn extra profits	• Resident volunteering	(2)

(continued)

Table 7.2 (continued)

Countermeasure	Operating body (name)	Operating body	Partner	Area of operation	Year of establishment	Outline of services	Classification by management	Source
• Mobile sales wagon	Fukui Co-operative Society	• Cooperative society		Hukui Pref.	2009	cooperative has its own logistical systems of non-shop retailing (i.e. a group purchase system and a home delivery system). By using its knowledge of its customers and distribution infrastructure, cooperative established suitable sources of goods for the mobile vending vehicle	• Business expansion	(2)
• Opening new shops	Yamoto	• Supermarket	• Local shops	Kofu City, Yamenashi Pref.	2011	A supermarket company sells its wholesale stock to individual local shops at cost price. Because of this support, local individual shops have increased their range of merchandise at low cost. As a result, local residents can enjoy shopping at nearby shops	• Business expansion • Cooperation with different industries	(2)

(continued)

Table 7.2 (continued)

Countermeasure	Operating body (name)	Operating body	Partner	Area of operation	Year of establishment	Outline of services	Classification by management	Source
• Shopping bus	Agle Bus Co.	• Bus company		Komakawa housing complex, Hidaka City, Saitama Pref.		This company has expanded its bus routes into poor food access areas and improved the accessibility of nearby grocery shops for local people	• Business expansion	(1)
• Mobile vending vehicle	Keio Corporation	• Railway company	• Municipality	Tama City and Hachioji City, Tokyo Pref.	2013	This railway company began a mobile vending vehicle service in residential complexes along its railway lines. The local government supports this service	• Entry from a different industry	Our own research
• Shopping bus	Aobadai community bus board of operation	• Local residents	• Municipality • Self-government association • Bus company	Aobadai District, Ichikawa City, Chiba Pref.		Ichikawa City has conducted a questionnaire survey of residents about the need for a shopping bus. Then Ichikawa city, neighborhood associations, and a consulting company held consultations and established a community bus service	• Resident volunteering • Cooperation with different industries	(2)

(continued)

Table 7.2 (continued)

	Countermeasure	Operating body (name)	Operating body	Partner	Area of operation	Year of establishment	Outline of services	Classification by management	Source
• Improving food access • Delivery	• Shopping services (shopping for an elderly person) • Shopping bus	Active Moco	• Rewards card service company	• Shopping Street Promotion Association	Some districts of Gotenba City, Susono City, Oyama Town and Hakone Town, Shizuoka Pref.	2011	This company offers a goods-delivery service and a shopping bus service to shops that use its point card system	• Entry from a different industry • Cooperation with different industries	(2)
	• Opening new shop • delivery	• Daikokuya Supermarket • Shimamoto Town Self-government Association	• Self-government Association	• Supermarket • Local residents	Wakayama Dai, Shimamoto Town, Osaka Pref.		A local supermarket in an old housing complex was closed due to the deterioration of its management. Therefore, residents made efforts to attract a new supermarket to their complex. To support the new supermarket, the residents established an NPO and started a home-delivery service for supermarket customers	• Resident volunteering	(1)
• Improving food access	• Mobile vending vehicle	Social welfare authority: Nijinokai	• Social welfare corporation	• User	Takashima City, Shiga Pref.	2011	This social welfare authority operates some mobile vending vehicles in rural areas. It also purchases wild vegetables from rural people and use them in a cafeteria managed by the social welfare authority	• Resident volunteering	(4)

(continued)

Table 7.2 (continued)

Countermeasure	Operating body (name)	Operating body	Partner	Area of operation	Year of establishment	Outline of services	Classification by management	Source
• Shopping bus	NPO corporation: KomyunitiZeene	• NPO	• Local residents	Fukushima City, Fukushima Pref.	2008	This NPO operates a courtesy bus service to a nearby supermarket. Many neighbors are financial members of this NPO and support the service. This bus service covers some expenses with advertising revenue. In addition, the NPO has a solar photoelectric generation system and gains extra income by selling electricity	• Resident volunteering	Our own research

Source (1) Ministry of Economy, Trade and Industry (2015) "Support manual for disadvantaged shoppers version 3.0" (Japanese) https://www.meti.go.jp/policy/economy/distribut ion/150427_manual_2.pdf (accessed January 2020) (Japanese); (2) Ministry of Economy, Trade and Industry (2011) "Support manual for disadvantaged shoppers version 2.0" (Japanese) http://warp.da.ndl.go.jp/info:ndljp/pid/8380059/www.meti.go.jp/policy/economy/distribution/manyuaruver2.pdf (accessed January 2020)(Japanese); (3) Kotani Yuichiro (2015) Food access issues and the address of Ministry of Agriculture, Forestry and Fisheries. Food industry for tomorrow. November 5–15. https://www.maff.go.jp/j/shokusan/eat/ pdf/nousui.pdf (accessed January 2020) (Japanese); (4) The Asahi newspaper, October 10, 2011 (A morning paper in Osaka area)

7.1.2 Classification by Management

It is impossible to sustain unprofitable businesses, even when they are useful for disadvantaged shoppers. Not only questions such as 'what kinds of services should we provide?' but also 'how should we provide services?' are important. Recently, some have noted this point and created new businesses. We have classified these new counter-measures[1] into seven types: Business Expansion (BE), Entry from a Different Industry (EDI), Co-operation with Different Industries (CDI), Resident Volunteering (RV), Co-operation with Industry, Government, Scholars, and the Local Community (CIGSLC), Welfare businesses (WBs), and New Businesses (NBs).[2] Below, we discuss the details of each type of service.

BE (Business Expansion) refers to disadvantaged shopper support services provided by companies whose main businesses relate to retailing and distribution. A typical example is the mobile vending vehicle service operated by a supermarket company. By expanding its main business, the company can implement FD counter-measures relatively easily. The company can utilize its know-how and corporate resources directly in its counter-measures, such as mobile vending vehicles. For example, a supermarket company can use its sales skills and merchandise supply system to provide a food vehicle service. This is the merit of BE. A co-operative society's sales vehicle service is a typical example of this type (see Sect. 7.2.1).

EDI (Entry from a Different Industry) is the business model whereby industries without a direct relationship with retailing and delivery derive some benefit by supporting disadvantaged shoppers. Although their main businesses are not retail or delivery, their business skills and resources are useful for operating disadvantaged shopper support services. Keio provides an example of an FD counter-measure. The Keio corporation is one of the largest private railway companies in Japan and it operates mobile sales vehicle businesses in housing complexes located along Keio's railway line (for more detail, see Sect. 7.2.2). The living environments of these housing complexes will be improved by this service. Moreover, the population in these areas is expected to increase (or at least to remain at current levels). The increased population will increase the number of rail passengers. Another example is Active Moco Ltd., which operates a rewards card service business in Gotenba city, Shizuoka prefecture. This company started a goods delivery service and a shopping bus service in 2011. These services are offered to shops that use Moco's point card system. If new customers are attracted by the delivery and shopping bus services, Moco's profits will also increase.

CDI (Co-operation with Different Industries) is a business model whereby different kinds of companies collaborate to promote support services for disadvantaged shoppers. For example, Japan Post and Yamato Transport are among the largest home delivery companies in Japan and they have nation-wide delivery networks. However, it is difficult for them to promote shopping support services alone. Therefore, they collaborate with local retailers and deliver their foods and goods to disadvantaged shoppers. Another remarkable case study is the association between Japan Agricultural Co-operatives (JA) and Yamazaki Baking. JA is a large organization that operates many supermarkets in agricultural villages. However, because of the rapid decrease of population in rural areas, some JA shops have lost considerable business. Yamazaki Baking is the largest breadmaking company in Japan. It not only manufactures a wide range of breads but also delivers them to many grocery shops around Japan via its own delivery networks. JA and Yamazaki co-operate to sustain rural JA shops (Yamazaki manages logistics and JA is responsible for retailing). They operate effectively and sustainably to offer a range of business resources and skills.

RV (Resident Volunteering) is a model whereby local people provide services to disadvantaged shoppers. Typical cases are grocery shop and shopping bus services managed by NPOs (non-profit organizations) established by local people in poor food access areas. In many cases, local people work without payment. Grocery shops of the 'Noson club' ('Noson' means 'agricultural village') in Nakatsu city, Oita prefecture, and 'Kurashi-kyodo Kan Nakayoshi' in Hitachinaka city, Ibaraki prefecture (see Sect. 7.2.3) are good examples of these. Shopping buses are also important services. Most bus services are operated by bus companies. However, these bus services are usually managed by councils that include representatives from local governments, bus companies, and local people. As mentioned in previous chapters, the main victims of FD issues are isolated elderly people who seldom accept support from strangers. On the other hand, neighbours, especially so-called 'local key people' such as the chairs of neighbourhood associations and local welfare commissioners, usually have good relationships of trust with these isolated elderly people. These elderly people tend to accept approaches from local people. Support from local people is necessary to promote aged welfare services. RV measures are superior in this respect. In addition, these volunteer activities often develop ties with neighbours (local social capital).

CIGSLC (Co-operation with Industry, Government, Scholars, and the Local Community) is a business model whereby private companies, the local government, academic researchers, and local people collaborate to address FD issues (through support services for disadvantaged shoppers). Collaborations with retailers, delivery companies, local communities, and municipalities facilitate the provision of a wide range of fresh foods to isolated elderly people at reasonable prices. If academic researchers join this collaboration and analyse municipality and company data on elderly people's living conditions, the precise distribution of elderly people who need care will be clear and predictable. These analyses would be useful to promote effective and sustainable measures. A good example is the mobile sales vehicle service in Ushiku city of Ibaraki prefecture (see Sect. 7.2.1). Although collaborations as described above remain rare in Japan, this type of management is necessary to resolve FD issues.

WBs (Welfare Businesses) are an advanced business model whereby a company provides welfare for aged people on behalf of local governments. A typical example is the Aikyo mobile vending vehicle service in the towns of Hino and Kofu in Tottori prefecture (see Sect. 7.2.4). The vehicles are operated by the Adachi company. This is a retail company based in the area. Aikyo provides the vehicle service and a safety confirmation service for elderly people, mobile medical treatment, a mobile library, and other services in Hino and Kofu towns. These services are unprofitable but necessary for elderly residents in the rural area. Therefore, municipalities position these services as social welfare. Aikyo has sufficient experience and management resources to provide the above services in this area, so the municipalities outsource these services to Aikyo through public subsidies.

NBs (New Businesses) are a new service model that departs from stereotypical support services. We discuss two case studies: *Onemile* and the Kurukuru Bus in Sects. 7.2.5 and 7.2.6 These companies directly pursue profitability and sustainability in support services and innovate new business models.

It is safe to say that the above six model types are attempts to establish profitable and sustainable support service models. In the next section, we introduce some remarkable case studies that offer possible solutions to FD issues. Although some case studies concern rural areas, the business models are also applicable to urban areas.

7.2 Remarkable Case Studies

7.2.1 [EB/CIGSLC] a Mobile Sales Vehicle Service Operated by an Alliance of Local People, Retailers, Government, and Scholars: Co-Op Hureai-Bin (Ushiku City, Ibaraki Prefecture)

The Ibaraki Co-op (co-operative) operates a mobile sales vehicle in Ushiku city, Ibaraki prefecture. This service is supported by a promotion committee composed of the Ibaraki Co-op, city council, the local social welfare council office, a local elderly care management centre, an NPO, and some town street neighbourhood associations. This service is a good example of the BE and CIGSLC models. We have already mentioned it in our previous book (Iwama 2011). Recently, we joined this council as scholars and analysed the prevailing FD issues in this city (we made FD maps and ascertained the potential need for a mobile vending vehicle) using a database offered by Ushiku city and the Ibaraki Co-op. We clarified who suffered from FDs, where they lived, and the difficulties they experienced in their daily lives. These are important pieces of information from which to develop sustainable and effective responses.

In this section, we show the outline and history of this mobile sales vehicle service. Ushiku is a small city located in the southern part of Ibaraki prefecture. Like other small Japanese towns, it is divided into an urban residential area and agricultural areas. Although there are many grocery shops including a co-op supermarket in the urban residential area, there are few grocery shops on the outskirts of the residential area or in the rural areas. Traditionally, this city's self-governing organizations are unified and very active. They established the Local Social Welfare Council in 2011. Generally, every city and town has a social welfare council. These councils are a public institution with many restrictions on their activities. On the other hand, a local social welfare council is a semi-governmental organization managed by local

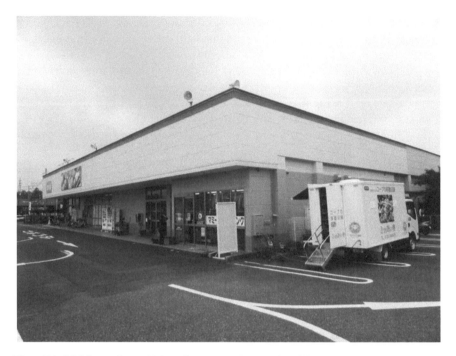

Photo 7.1 Mobile vending vehicle at Co-op store (Ushiku City, 2014, taken by Iwama)

communities (self-governing associations). A local social welfare council can act more vigorously and independently than public councils. The Ibaraki Co-op began mobile vending services in March 2012 (Photo 7.1). The vehicle has a 1.5t track, which has been improved to carry fresh foods and frozen/refrigerated foods (Photo 7.2). This vehicle can carry about 350–400 items. This service is supported by the promotion committee. The route starts at the co-op supermarket and travels mainly around the city.

This vehicle has a remarkable feature to secure a customer base. It is not only a vehicle but a place for cultural exchanges between local residents. Bus stops are sited in open spaces. Many shoppers (mainly elderly people and young mothers with babies) enjoy shopping and chatting with neighbours. This is a good opportunity for young mothers to obtain useful advice from elderly people who have much experience of childcare (Photo 7.3). This service also provides a good opportunity to ensure the safety of seniors. Ibaraki Co-op sometimes holds food education classes at some bus stops.

Each bus stop is managed by local residents. Generally, the leaders or welfare commissioners in each neighbourhood manage bus stops. They are the so-called local key people and know all about their neighbours' situations, such as who is shut in at home and isolated from society and who has difficulty going shopping. When the mobile sales vehicle comes to their bus stop, the bus stop managers invite

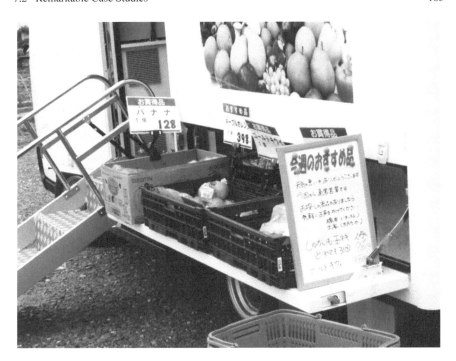

Photo 7.2 Wide range of fresh foods (Ushiku City, 2014, taken by Iwama)

isolated elderly people and disadvantaged shoppers (Photo 7.4). Generally, community leaders and welfare commissioners have good relationships of trust with elderly neighbours. This is why many elderly people accept the invitation and enjoy shopping from the vehicle. This support from local key people enables the Ibaraki Co-op to operate the mobile sales vehicle effectively.

Recently, the promotion committee co-operated with researchers and clarified the FD issues in Ushiku city. Previously, no one knew who was in FDs and where they lived. FD maps helped to improve the mobile vending vehicle service. Many vehicle services operated around Japan, but many operators do not know their target markets. Therefore, many such initiatives go bankrupt within a few years of the service starting. As in the Ushiku case study, academic analyses are necessary to develop sustainable interventions.

In Ushiku city, owing to the co-operation between various committees, the council manages the sales vehicle service effectively (Fig. 7.1). The most difficult aspect of these measures is to attract customers. Support from government and local people makes it possible to overcome this difficulty. However, even though the business concerns an aspect of social welfare, the government cannot support specific companies' business activities. If the business is operated by the council, the government may support it. In addition, FDs are invisible and difficult to identify and locate, but researchers can overcome this difficulty.

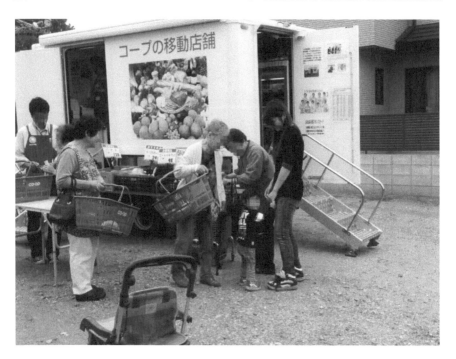

Photo 7.3 Shopping scenery (Ushiku City, 2014, taken by Iwama)

Table 7.3 shows the history of Ushiku's vehicle service. It is safe to say that this co-operative initiative was achieved by the following four factors. First is the residents' strong solidarity and initiative. Before the vehicle service started, many neighbour-hood communities operated their own voluntary services, but few performed well. From these experiences, neighbourhood communities learned how important and difficult shopping support services are to manage. Therefore, when Ibaraki Co-op and Ushiku city council invited neighbourhood communities, many accepted the invitation gladly.

The second factor is the existence of local social welfare councils. Public social welfare councils are a kind of public association based on the *Social Welfare Act* and they are virtually prohibited to support specific companies' activities. However, local councils are both public and private and can support these companies' activities. In addition, local councils have strong connections with local neighbourhood associations. Therefore, local councils can pressure neighbourhood associations into supporting measures to address FDs.

The third factor is the local government's rapid responses. The mayor thought highly of Ibaraki Co-op's vending vehicle project and strongly supported it. He showed strong leadership and invited many organizations concerned with elderly people's welfare to a promotion committee for the vending vehicle service. The first round-table conference was hold in January 2011. In this conference, the parties decided to collaborate to support this service. In addition, they added other

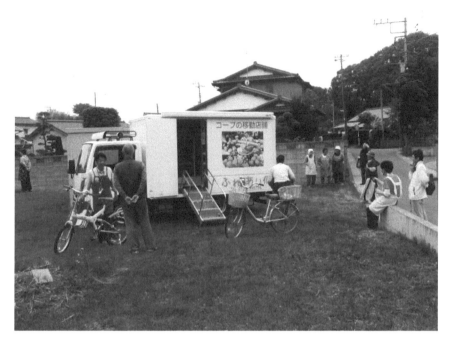

Photo 7.4 Bus stop manager (in front of the vehicle) and shoppers (Ushiku City, 2014, taken by Iwama)

members and formed the Ushiku City Shopping Support/Urban Development Promotion Committee. Then they started a vending vehicle service in Ushiku city. At that stage, the support system for disadvantaged shoppers was established. In addition, the city council included the Department of Social Welfare, the Department of Health Management, the Department of Urban Planning, the Department of Commerce and Tourism, and the Department of the Civic Life. This collaborative arrangement soon fully supported the vending vehicle service. Moreover, the parties fully supported our research on FD issues in this city. Thanks to their co-operation, we could conduct interviews and distribute a large-scale questionnaire survey.

The fourth factor is the devoted efforts of retail companies. nine years have passed since Ibaraki Co-op began its mobile sales vehicle service in Mito city (the capital city of Ibaraki prefecture) in February 2011. Although the number of customers has increased, Ibaraki Co-op could not gain sufficient profits from this business. The Japanese government offered to subsidize this initiative, but Ibaraki Co-op does not receive any subsidies from the government and bears all the costs of the vending vehicle service itself. Although the company promotes healthy eating for elderly people through this service, it must be remembered that almost all disadvantaged shopper support services in Japan are built on these companies' efforts and self-sacrifice.

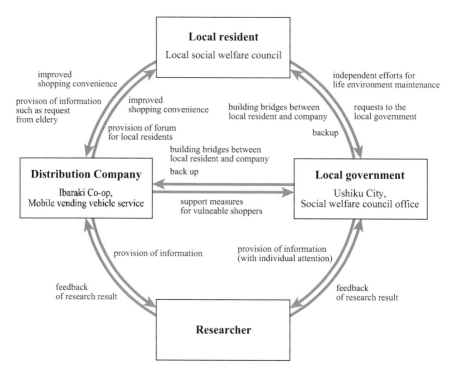

Fig. 7.1 Co-operation between various committees, the council manages the sales vehicle service. *Source* Iwama ed. (2017)

7.2.2 [EDI] a Railway Company Mobile Vending Vehicle at Tama New Town

One afternoon, there was almost no traffic in the Matsugaya housing complex in Tama New Town. A mobile vending vehicle arrived at 14:00, and people began to gather. When two salespeople began preparing to sell their goods, about 10 customers gathered before the product display and cash register preparations were completed (Photo 7.5). When sales began, commodities such as vegetables and fruits sold steadily. Some shoppers talked to acquaintances. Shoppers were uninterrupted and the staff had no time to rest until sales were completed. When the allotted time was up, the vending vehicle left for the next place. This is how the Keio Corporation mobile vending vehicle operates.

In Tama New Town in the western part of Tokyo, there are areas where retail shops have closed, and the shopping environment is deteriorating. Ito-Yokado and Keio operate vending vehicles there. Ito-Yokado began its service in July 30, 2013, and Keio began its service in November 25, 2013. This section introduces the mobile vending vehicle service in the suburbs of large cities, focusing on the Keio service.

Table 7.3 Development of cooperation between local government, companies and residents in Ushiku's mobile vending vehicle service

Before 2011	• Leaders of neighborhood associations had an interest in disadvantaged shopper issues. They researched how to support these residents
February 2011	• Ibaraki Co-op started a mobile vending vehicle service in Mito City, the capital city of Ibaraki Pref.
	• Neighborhood associations have established local social welfare councils.[*1]
	• These councils started disadvantaged shopper support services as joint enterprises → As a result, they realized the difficulty of operating these services by themselves
June 2011	• Representatives of Ushiku Social Welfare Council visited the cooperative's mobile vending vehicle service. They reported the findings of the observational visits to local social welfare councils
	• Ibaraki Co-op planed to start a new vending vehicle service in Ushiku City and it asked Ushiku City to support the service
	• The mayor of Ushiku City accepted the cooperative's offer (The mayor had previous experience in the mobile vending vehicle business. Therefore, he know well that this business was not profitable and difficult to maintain without support from government)
January 2012	• The mayor of Ushiku City, chief director of Ibaraki Co-op, and chief director of Ushiku Social Welfare Council met to discuss a disadvantaged shopper support service. They decided to collaborate. Ushiku Social Welfare Council played an intermediary role in this meeting
May 2012	• Ushiku City, Ushiku Social Welfare Council, a community general support center, neighborhood associations (local social welfare councils), an NPO (a transfer service) and the Ibaraki Co-op concluded an agreement. They established a committee to promote the mobile vending vehicle service
	• Ushiku City promotes public support for this support service. In short, they made a multi-agency office composed of the Social Welfare Division, Health Management Division, Urban Planning Division, Commerce and Tourism Division, and Division for Volunteering Support Policy. This cross-organizational office comprehensively supports the cooperative's activities
	• **Ibaraki Co-op started operating a mobile vending vehicle service in Ushiku City**
July 2012	• Ibaraki Prefecture adopted this disadvantaged shopper support service as a "new public proposal model" project in 2012
August 2012	• A promotion committee held the "Ushiku roundtable discussion" with concerned parties and discussed shopping support services and life services for elderly people
January 2014	• The researchers carried out a large-scale questionnaire survey of all residents with full support from Ushiku City (Senior Citizens' Welfare Division, and Health Management Division)
March 2015	• The researchers held a briefing session and shared survey results with a promotion committee for the mobile vending vehicle service

Source Interview survey

[*1]Local social welfare councils are subordinate organizations of the Ushiku Social Welfare Council. The Ushiku Social Welfare Council is a kind of public organization. To establish local subordinate organizations, neighborhood associations can obtain public support for their social welfare activities from local government

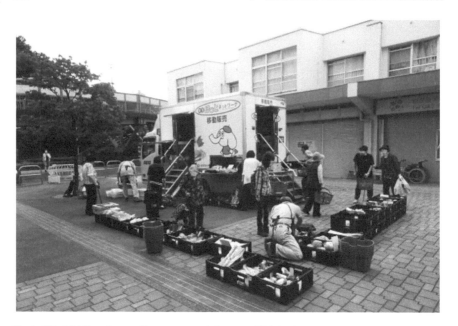

Photo 7.5 Mobile sales vending wagon and shoppers (2015, taken by Ikeda)

Why is Keio, a railway company, operating a mobile vending vehicle? Keio needs to attract railway passengers. Therefore, it is developing a service business for residents living along the Keio line and aims to increase the value of their residences by solving their problems. One such service is the mobile vending vehicle.

The details of this mobile sales business are as follows. Keio uses a two-ton vehicle modified for mobile sales. The rear and sides of the vehicle are open so that shoppers can access it and select goods to buy. The vehicle has a refrigerator in which chilled items are displayed, and room-temperature items are displayed around the vehicle in containers (Photo 7.5). There are a wide range of goods on the vehicle, including fresh foods such as meat, fish, vegetables, and fruits, refrigerated products such as milk and eggs, processed foods, seasonings, and daily necessities such as toilet paper. More than 400 items are on the vehicle. The sales staff report that fresh vegetables and fruits sell well. The price of the commodities is the same as that in the Keio shop, except for vegetables. In general, two or three sales people staff the vehicle.

The daily schedule of mobile sales is as follows (Table 7.4). The mobile vending vehicle makes four stops per day from Monday to Friday. In the morning, at the Takahata Keio shop, commodities are loaded on the vehicle. The vehicle goes to two sales stops in the morning before returning to the shop once to replenish its supplies, then it makes another two stops in the afternoon. In the evening, some products (vegetables, meat, fish, chilled food, and expired goods) are returned to the shop.

About 90% of customers at this mobile service are women, many o f them elderly; there are also women in their 30–40 s and mothers with infants. The average number of shoppers per day is about 80. The average value of sales per customer is just under

Table 7.4 Schedule of mobile sales in 2015

08:15	Commodities are loaded onto the wagon at Keio shop
09:30	Departure to first stop
10:10–10:45	Wagon sells its items at its first stop
	Wagon moves to second stop
11:20–11:55	Wagon sells its items at second stop
12:30	Wagon returns to the shop and replenishes supplies
13:30	Wagon moves to third stop
14:15–14:50	Wagon sells its items at the third stop
	Wagon moves to fourth stop
15:25–16:00	Wagon sells its items at fourth stop
16:30	Wagon return to shop. Staff members return unsold goods.

Source Keio in-house document

1,200 yen (about 11USD), but it varies because some buy a little of what they lack and others buy all the food they need. The value of daily sales per stop is about 25,000 yen, and the total value is less than 100,000 yen.

Since December 2015, the Keio mobile sales business has been in the red. However, the objective was to improve the value of residences along the line, so Keio is not concerned about its profitability. Keio does not intend to withdraw from the mobile sales business because it makes a loss, but it is considering improving profitability by reconsidering its sales locations.

Regarding the difficulties of establishing a mobile sales business, Keio makes the following two points. First, it is not known whether the vehicle will attract customers unless it actually starts mobile sales. Even if the mobile vending vehicle stops at places without supermarkets or convenience shops nearby, it may not attract shoppers. Some stops are no longer used because there were too few shoppers. In other words, it is difficult to identify people having trouble shopping in advance. For this reason, mobile sales are difficult.

The other difficulty is securing a suitable place to sell. When Keio decides on a place for mobile sales, candidate places are listed based on the number of nearby households and the location of supermarkets and convenience shops. However, it may not be possible to sell at a candidate place. The first issue is parking a two-ton vehicle, and the second is obtaining permission to do so.

Keio obtained the permission of Hachioji City and Tama City to park the vending vehicle at suitable places. For example, Hachioji city provided a letter of recommendation for permission to park in a housing complex. In addition, Hachioji city negotiated for permission from the district organization for the vehicle to conduct mobile sales in the shopping street. In this way, Hachioji city has played a major role in securing a place for mobile sales.

As the case of Keio shows, the problem for mobile sales in urban areas is to secure a place to park the vehicle, and it is important to obtain the co-operation of local governments and local residents.

7.2.3 [RV] Grocery Shop Managed by Residents—The Kurashi-Kyodo Kan Nakayoshi NPO (Hitachi-Naka City, Ibaraki Prefecture)

It is very difficult for public service workers and retailers to persuade elderly people to improve their shopping and eating habits. However, if key local trusted people approach them, elderly people often attempt to change their habits. Here, we introduce the Kurashi-Kyodo Kan Nakayoshi NPO initiative as a good example of an RV measure to address FDs. Nakayoshi is an NPO that has repurposed a closed co-op shop to offer a wide range of fresh foods, a restaurant, a café, and other facilities to local residents. This shop is staffed by volunteers. According to a 2014 survey (Yakushiji 2015), 74.7% of all residents over the age of 65 years in this neighbourhood use this popular shop. We described this initiative in our previous book (Iwama 2011). In this book, we outline this measure and describe the new activities undertaken since 2011.

Nakayoshi is in Hitachi-naka City, Ibaraki Prefecture. This shop is located in a large housing complex 10 min' drive from the main train station (Photo 7.6). This is a typical industrial city built around Hitachi Ltd., a global industrial corporation. There are many factories and workers' housing complexes in this city. Many of these housing complexes, including that of Nakayoshi, were built during the so-called 'Japanese high economic growth period' during the late 1950s to early 1970s. Now, many residents are over 65 years old. In these housing complexes, many grocery shops and banks closed in the 1990s. Even the co-op's medium-sized supermarket closed in May 2004 because it was making a loss. Local people thought that 'without a nearby grocery shop, many elderly people will have difficulty shopping. Therefore, we must do something to maintain our living environment'. Local unionists for the co-op shop established a review board and discussed the refurbishment of the shop facilities. They then distributed a questionnaire to gather local residents' opinions and found that many were very concerned about the lack of nearby grocery shops. In addition, the residents requested not only shopping facilities and restaurants, but also hobby clubs, sports clubs, cultural schools, and other organizations. The most serious problem was recruiting volunteers. The members of the review board had little experience in retailing; thus, they did not believe they could earn sufficient profit to hire shop staff on regular salaries. Therefore, the review board recruited local residents as volunteers. About 60 people applied for this volunteer work. In addition, the review board established a trial market during the day. This reaped about 20,000 yen per day, which is not a huge sum of money, but was sufficient to run a volunteer grocery shop. Thus, they established an NPO named 'Kurashi Kyodo-Kan

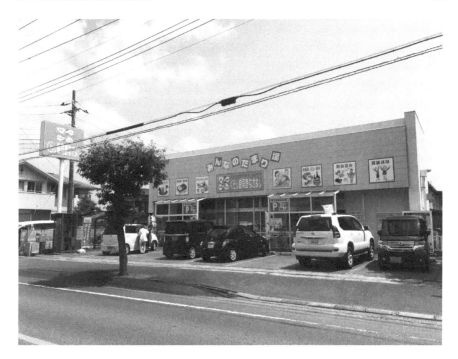

Photo 7.6 Kurashi-Kyodo Kan Nakayoshi (Hitachinaka City, 2020, taken by Iwama)

Nakayoshi' in 2005 and opened the Nakayoshi ('friends') shop on the site of the former co-op supermarket.

Since this shop opened, a large supermarket and a convenience shop have also opened in this area; therefore, the poor food access issue has been resolved to some degree. However, the number of Nakayoshi customers has not decreased.

The total floor space at Nakayoshi is about 330.6 m^2 and is divided into partitions (Photo 7.7). This shop sells not only a range of fresh foods, but also some hand-made daily meals, breads, processed foods, frozen foods, flavour enhancers, and other products. Although the range of goods is limited, customers can purchase popular ingredients to cook healthy meals. In addition, Nakayoshi offers some hobby clubs (e.g., cultural clubs, an exercise class for elderly people, a health class, and a cookery class), childcare services, after-school care for children, among other services (Table 7.5).

Nakayoshi's activities are staffed by volunteers. The heaviest work is cooking daily meals. Unusually, Nakayoshi pays cooks 260 yen per hour. The minimum guaranteed wage under Japanese law was 849 yen per hour in 2019; therefore, 260 yen is not a salary but an allowance for heavy work. Other volunteers work without an allowance, but many residents continue to apply for positions. They are all smiles and work energetically at Nakayoshi. Several staff members manage the affairs of the organization, but in general the management of each department has been left to the volunteers' discretion. If trouble arises, the volunteers contribute ideas and discuss

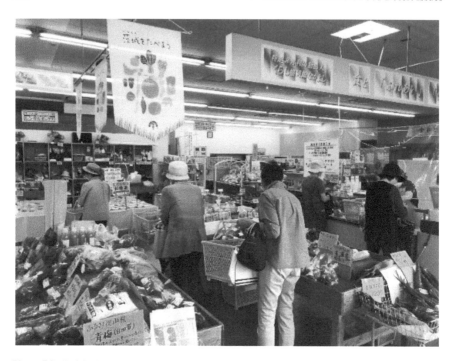

Photo 7.7 Inside the store (Hitachinaka City, 2020, taken by Iwama)

Table 7.5 Business operations in Nakayoshi in 2015

Name	Kurashi-Kyodo Kan Nakayoshi NPO initiative	
Number of staff members		
	Regular members	91
	Support members	285
Total floor space		
	330.6 m^2	
Number of users		
	Total	81,963
	Shopping, restaurant and café	63,184
Business operations		
	Food retailing	
	Restaurant and café	
	Hobby clubs (cultural school, sports club, health class, cooking class, etc.)	
	Child care	
	Annual events	
	Free after-school child care class	

Source Annual Report of Nakayoshi (2020)

Table 7.6 Number of users in Nakayoshi in 2015 (%)

	Total	<50 years old	51–64 years old	65–74 years old	>75 years old
Purchase of foods	61.0	50.0	64.3	58.2	68.9
Purchase of meals	39.9	25.0	42.9	39.0	40.5
Restaurant and café	17.3	8.3	8.6	16.9	28.4
Hobby club	21.7	8.3	14.3	24.3	25.7
Annual events	15.2	25.0	12.9	13.0	21.6
Health class	8.0	0.0	1.4	10.2	10.8
Dinner parties	3.6	0.0	1.4	1.7	10.8
Others	3.3	16.7	1.4	1.7	6.8
Nothing	25.3	41.7	24.3	28.8	14.9

Source Yakushiji ed. (2015)

them together. They then decide how to resolve the problem. The staff members do not seek money but a purpose in life and mutual aid. We believe that this is the reason they work hard and with a smile, which is the most remarkable feature of Nakayoshi.

Nakayoshi has 91 regular members and 285 supporting members. Many live in the housing complex. It has 81,963 customers per year with 265 per day (as reported from the 2015 general meeting). The number of users has increased since 2009, when the figures reported in our previous book were gathered (Iwama 2011). Our 2014 questionnaire survey showed that many elderly people used Nakayoshi for various purposes, such as shopping, hobby clubs, and meetings with neighbours (Table 7.6). Staff and users of Nakayoshi often overlap. In short, Nakayoshi is a place where local residents support each other. Since its establishment, the number of users has increased, and the business has remained in the black. An active balance of payments has been maintained even after the opening of a competing supermarket and some convenience shops in the neighbourhood. This means that Nakayoshi offers something more valuable to the local residents than a simple shopping centre.

How does Nakayoshi maintain its profitability and sustainability? We propose the following four successful factors to answer this question.

The first factor is the creation of an attractive workplace environment where volunteers can work hard. As mentioned above, all staff members are unpaid, yet they willingly work hard. In general, organizations pay their employees as compensation for their labour. If an organization does not pay its workers, it will become very difficult to maintain operations. However, Nakayoshi pays its staff in something other than salaries and it runs smoothly. It is very difficult to explain clearly what Nakayoshi pays volunteers instead of money. Phrases like 'purpose in life' or the 'pleasure of dedication' are insufficient to describe the compensation for volunteer workers. However, we can see this intangible compensation when we visit Nakayoshi and see the smiles on the faces of customers and volunteers.[3]

The second factor is the use of local human resources. Volunteers have special skills such as cooking, management, clerical work, trades, calligraphy, tea ceremony, storytelling, and traditional Japanese games, which elderly adults have cultivated through the course of their long lives. Nakayoshi asks volunteers to do what they want to do; therefore, the staff members choose their volunteer work according to their special skills and experiences. People with good cooking skills often cook. Likewise, some people teach calligraphy or the tea ceremony, while others work in the management division. The volunteers use their special skills for Nakayoshi. This scheme gives elderly people a sense of fulfilment and purpose in life.

The third factor is the support from local people. Many people do not participate in the initiative, but they support Nakayoshi indirectly. Some people join as supporting members and pay an annual membership fee. Some people enjoy shopping or participating in hobby club activities there. In addition, much equipment, such as dishes, tables, and electric pianos, are donated by local people.

The fourth factor is the co-operation with local farmers and companies. Nakayoshi has a policy of supporting local industries and trades with many local farmers and companies (such as a dairy, a tofu seller, a sushi restaurant, a butcher shop, a fishmonger's, and a coffee supplier). In addition, Nakayoshi sells a wide range of goods, including breads, sweets, bottled foods, and handcrafted goods made by the local community workshop. Moreover, Nakayoshi has consignment sale contracts with local farmers and food producers. Consignment sales contracts are a sales method whereby wholesalers and manufacturers consign foods to retailers (in this case, Nakayoshi) and pay a commission fee to retailers. The compounding fee is decided in proportion to the total sales of goods. Under this contract, Nakayoshi has a right to return unsold goods to the wholesalers. Therefore, Nakayoshi can avoid the risk of dead stock. However, Nakayoshi attempts to reduce dead stock by sharing sales information (the rate at which goods are sold) with wholesalers and improving its inventory control and sales predictions. If fresh food is unsold, Nakayoshi purchases much of it to use in daily meals. Thus, Nakayoshi manages its business in co-operation with local farmers and companies.

Recently, consumption trends have changed. On the one hand, as society ages, the total sales of fresh foods are decreasing. On the other hand, the demand for daily meals and cafés/restaurants is increasing because many elderly people do not want to cook for themselves every day. The total sales of fresh food in 2015 was 96.5% compared with those in 2014. However, the total sales of daily meals (100.7%) and café/restaurant meals (104.2%) are going well. Daily meals are in high demand. However, Nakayoshi's cooks are also aging. To cook a large amount of food every day is arduous for aged cooks. How should Nakayoshi develop its organizational framework to adapt to population aging? This is important. For the exercise classes and hobby clubs, the number of participants has increased compared with last year (exercise class, 136%; hobby clubs, 105%).

Socio-economic conditions are also changing. In tandem with population aging, the number of vacant houses is increasing in the housing complex where Nakayoshi is located. Recently, young householders have gradually moved into these vacant houses or adjacent public housing. Some are low-income families, including single mothers. In this situation, Nakayoshi's staff members have found some children who do not eat enough at home for many reasons. The residents of this housing complex used to be relatively wealthy, and childhood poverty was not yet obvious. Nakayoshi has offered a children's cafeteria offering free food to poor children since 2015. In addition, it has a free after-school childcare class. In this class, local elderly people and children play traditional Japanese games together. Sometimes, elderly people also help children with their homework. About ten children visit Nakayoshi every day. Nakayoshi noticed these new problems quickly and responded efficiently. For this flexible response, Nakayoshi deserves special recognition. Recently, some local high school students joined the activities at Nakayoshi to support the children's cafeteria and the free after-school childcare class. The local government highly values these activities, which were commissioned as government projects in 2019.

The coronavirus disease 2019 (COVID-19) pandemic has impacted Nakayoshi's activities significantly in 2020. At the time of writing, it is not clear whether the pandemic is a transient or permanent problem. Therefore, we shall consider Nakayoshi's present situation after the pandemic and the previous trend separately. Table 7.7 shows a profile of Nakayoshi for the period between June 2019 and May 2020. Nakayoshi added seven regular members but lost 10 support members between 2015 and 2020. The number of users is also decreasing rapidly. The main reason for these decreases is the temporary suspension of hobby club activities. Since March 2020, Nakayoshi has stopped all hobby club activities and closed a restaurant and café. Although the free after-school child-care class and the children's cafeteria remain open, numbers of users are limited. Before the COVID-19 pandemic, many hobby club participants enjoyed shopping at Nakayoshi before or after club activities. Following the loss of these customers, sales of food and meals have fallen rapidly. However, the number of customers purchasing daily food (not participants in club activities) has increased slightly. Many of these customers are so-called poor

Table 7.7 Business operations in Nakayoshi in 2020

Name	Kurashi-Kyodo Kan Nakayoshi NPO initiative
Number of staff members	
Regular members	98
Support members	275
Total floor space	
330.6 m^2	
Number of users	
Total	74,610
Shopping, restaurant and café	53,346
Business operations	
Food retailing	
Children's cafeteria	
Free after-school child care class	

Source Annual report of Nakayoshi (2020)

food-access elderly people without private cars. They are deemed to be vulnerable in the COVID-19 pandemic and they really appreciate the existence of nearby grocery stores (such as Nakayoshi). The problem is that almost all Nakayoshi's volunteer staff are also older and have a high risk of catching COVID-19. Nevertheless, no volunteers have quit. They pay close attention to infection prevention and continue to work at Nakayoshi. However, for the first time since its establishment, Nakayoshi's finances have dipped into the red in this period. If the pandemic continues for a long time, it will be very difficult to maintain Nakayoshi's activities.

7.2.4 [WB] an Innovative Approach by a Mobile Supermarket Business: Adachi Company (Hino Town and Kofu Town, Tottori Prefecture)

The Aikyo mobile vending vehicle, operated by the Adachi Company, visits a total of 70 communities in two mountain towns. Aikyo's mobile vending vehicle has been described in a case study in previous books (Iwama 2011, 2013). It is an innovative project designed to help those who have limited access to shops. A previous survey conducted in 2010 found that the population in areas where Aikyo operates is decreasing by approximately 100 annually (Iwama 2011). It was pointed out that it would be difficult for the mobile vending vehicle to continue operating independently. Thereafter, a follow-up survey was conducted, which found that the supermarket had launched new business plans, such as collaborating with the public sector and participating in local government welfare projects for older people. This section begins with a brief reflection on work to date by the Aikyo mobile vending vehicle and subsequently discusses its current transition to a new business model.

Adachi is a grocery company that operates four supermarkets and the Lawson convenience shop franchise shops in Hino and Kofu towns, Hino-gun, and Tottori. The company also sells products in remote local areas through its mobile vending vehicle. Hino-gun is located in the Chugoku Mountains, in south-western Tottori Prefecture. Hino-gun consists of the following three towns: Nichinan, Hino, and Kofu. In 2015, the total population of the three towns was approximately 11,600. At over 40%, the proportion of people aged over 65 years in the towns is high. The towns are quintessential examples of isolated mountain villages. Not only the grocery shops and restaurants in the villages, but also all of the Japan Agricultural Co-operative shops, which sold groceries and daily necessities have closed down in 1994. In 2010, there were only 19 grocery shops in the area, including those of Adachi. Aikyo has the only supermarket in Kofu.

The Adachi Company was founded by Mr. Kyoji Adachi, who used to work for the local consumers' co-op, which went bankrupt. Adachi took over the old shop buildings of the co-op and started a new business with his older colleagues (Sakamoto 2010; Seki 2015). The business focuses on the local community and aims to address the needs of local people. In 1993, the business launched a mobile vending vehicle project with the aim of helping older people who did not have their own cars to go shopping (Table 7.8, Photo 7.8). Such older adults have a particularly hard time in winter because the mountainous area is covered with thick snow. We described the details of the mobile vending vehicle in the prior paper; therefore, we will not repeat them in this section. Aikyo not only operates the mobile vending vehicle but also orders items that are not in stock on behalf of their customers upon request. Additionally, the Adachi Company collaborates with the Tottori prefectural government in a community safety watch program. It has also undertaken the task of

Table 7.8 History of Adachi Company

Year	Business
1990	Aikyo is founded (the former cooperative shop in Hino Town is used)
1993	A mobile supermarket is established with a one-tone vehicle
2004	Aikyo takes over JA's closed-down shop and some of its employees It opens three shops in Kofu Town
2005	Aikyo takes over an additional closed JA shop and opens the second shop in Hino Town
2008	The Lawson Kofu Town shop is opened (the first mobile vending vehicle in Japan that sells the products of a convenience store)
	An agreement for watching over and protecting people in mountainous areas, entitled *A project to support activities for monitoring and protecting mountainous villages*, was made with Tottori Pref.
2009	*The Protecting the Lives of those in Mountainous Communities in Tottori joint project* grant was awarded by Tottori Pref.
	The Emergency Support Project for Areas Where Seniors Have Limited Access to Shops in Kofu Town grant was awarded by Kofu Town
2010	One shop in Kofu Town is closed down
	Joint sales of products for people with disabilities is undertaken by a welfare service center
2011	The Nursing Delivery Services project is established through collaboration with Hino Hospital
2012	*The Community-Inclusive Shopping Service Validation Project* grant is awarded by Kofu and Hino Towns
2014	*The Hino Town Community-Inclusive Shopping Service Project* grant is awarded by Hino Town
	Personalized mobile shop services are established through collaboration with the Hino Chamber of Commerce
	Mobile library services are established through collaboration with Hino Town Library
2017	Mr. Adachi transferred some parts of his business to a successor (a former colleague)
2020	A rapid increase in patronage of the mobile vending vehicle because of the COVID-19 virus

Source Interviews and the Support manual for disadvantaged shoppers version 3.0 by the Ministry of Economy, Trade and Industry

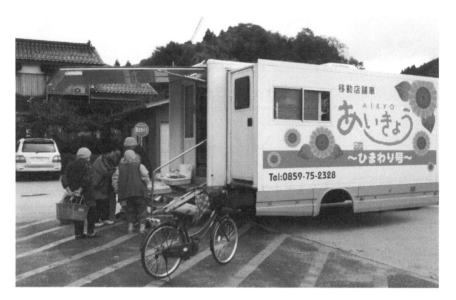

Photo 7.8 Senior users of the mobile vending vehicle (Kofu town, 2010, taken by Sasaki)

checking that older people are safe at home as part of the local government welfare service programme (Photo 7.9).

The previous paper summarized the factors that make it possible for Adachi Company to continue operating its mobile vending vehicle in the mountainous Kofu town, where the population continues to decline. The factors that we pointed out were these: the structure of the town, where scattered villages are located within a 15-minute drive from the town centre as well as an efficient delivery system, and a strong, mutually dependent relationship between the shop and its customers.

Despite a decrease in the local population of approximately 500 from the last survey, Adachi has made noteworthy progress with a new business model. The company began providing services through collaboration with the public sector in 2011 (Table 7.7). As Seki (2015) has pointed out, Adachi's business has become increasingly community oriented. The company signed a collaboration agreement with the prefecture for a safety watch program for older people in 2008 and has undertaken a community-inclusive shopping program from the local government. Following these transitions, the company also started the following projects: the Nursing Delivery Service in collaboration with Hino Hospital, a local public hospital, in 2011; personalized mobile shop services with the Hino Chamber of Commerce in 2014; and the Mobile Library Service with the Hino Town Library in 2014.

The Nursing Delivery Service commenced in July 2011. Under this business model, a vehicle from Hino Hospital accompanies the mobile vending vehicle and hospital staff provide health consultation services to local older adult shoppers. The collaboration was realized because the head nurse of Hino Hospital became interested in Adachi's work. Two nurses and one nationally registered dietitian visit Hino

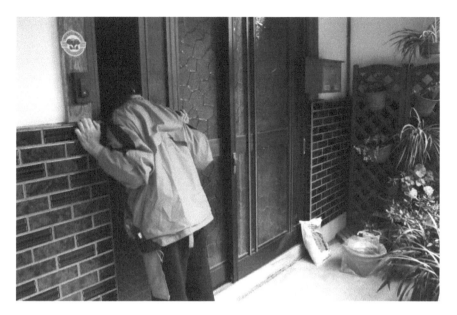

Photo 7.9 Communication between staff and local seniors (a safety watch program) (Kofu town, 2010, taken by Sasaki)

and Kofu towns once every two months. They visit the former in even-numbered months and the latter in odd months. During each visit, they provide various health-related services, such as measuring blood pressure, announcing the schedule for outpatient appointments at the hospital, and giving health advice. These services are well received by the local community and a large number of older adults use them.

Meanwhile, personalized mobile shop services offered by the Hino Chamber of Commerce commenced in August 2014. They were started as a pilot project and designed to validate a sustainable community support system in the mountainous areas of Tottori. According to documents from the Hino Chamber of Commerce, the aim of the services is to identify a new sales channel for products that are not sold by Aikyo, as well as product development. Aikyo's mobile vending vehicle has a total of six routes. One member of the casual staff of the Hino Chamber of Commerce accompanies the mobile vending vehicle on one of the six routes every weekday and hears customers' requests (Photo 7.10). A survey in November 2015 found that four to five orders for items such as soil and fertilizers are placed weekly with personalized mobile shop services.

Additionally, the Mobile Library Service was started in September 2014 in collaboration with a local library. A vehicle from the library accompanies the mobile vending vehicle so that supermarket customers can also borrow books from the library (Photo 7.11). Not only older people with limited transportation and physical disabilities but also others use the Mobile Library Service because they appreciate convenience. They do not have to travel to the town centre to use the library and can

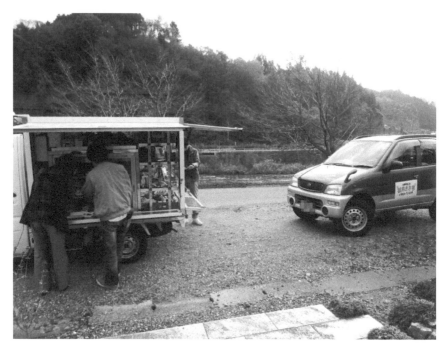

Photo 7.10   A vehicle of Aikyo's mobile supermarket (left) and a car from the HinoChamber of Commerce providing personalized mobile store services (right) (Hino Town, 2015, taken by Sasaki)

borrow books when they shop at the mobile vending vehicle. Books can be returned either to the Mobile Library or to the library in the town, adding further convenience to this service. In 2014, Hino Town Library conducted a questionnaire survey in all areas visited by Aikyo's mobile vending vehicle, with the aim of identifying villages with high demand. The library has its normal operations and holds events. It currently has two routes (five stops on each route) and runs once a month. The number of users of the Mobile Library Service fluctuates depending on the weather and the agricultural cycle. Notwithstanding this, at least six to seven people use the Mobile Library each time. During the seven-month period from September to March in the 2014 financial year, 173 people used the service. Hino Town Library has expanded its mobile services. It also started offering mobile library services at public facilities and opened borrowing stations (Yoraiya Library) in remote villages at around the same time as it started collaborating with Adachi. Our interview survey of the library found that they considered that there was a demand for library services from one-third of the local residents. The library is considering accompanying Aikyo's mobile vending vehicle more frequently in future.

   As described above, Aikyo's mobile vending vehicle has become the hub of local public and private services for older people in remote communities in various areas from food, health, welfare, and entertainment to shopping. As we have indicated elsewhere, this has been achieved because the Adachi mobile vending vehicle effectively

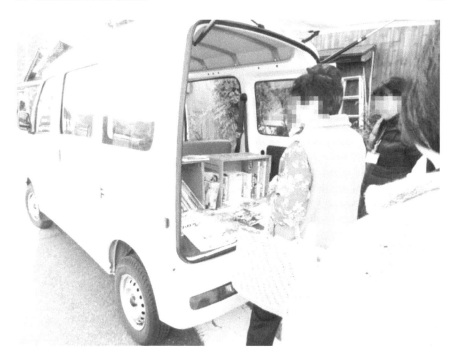

Photo 7.11 Seniors choosing books to borrow at the mobile library prior to shopping (Hino Town, 2015, taken by Sasaki)

services approximately 70 communities in the two towns. Tottori prefecture has set up a grant program, called the Community-Inclusive Shopping program (Kaimono Fukushi Service). This reflects the fact that shopping is considered an integral part of welfare services by members of the community.

Against a backdrop of an increasing older population in a shrinking community in its business area, it is clear that Adachi is currently shifting its business model to a semi-public one by collaborating with governments and the public sector. With a deep knowledge of all communities in its business area, Adachi is complementing the welfare function of the local government. As a result, the company offsets losses from its retail business. Moreover, the company is currently building a 'mobile-oriented' system centred on the mobile vending vehicle through collaboration with public sectors to support local residents in their daily lives.

Adachi stated that the company's business model is feasible because it operates across small communities over a small area. Adachi and his colleagues are deeply connected to the community and have a track record of contributing to it. Moreover, they have few competitors in the area. These factors may have enabled Aikyo to gain the trust of the community. Despite it being a private company, Adachi has built a partnership with the local government to provide various public services. A large number of local services have shrunk or been cancelled, and the local government has faced difficulties in providing necessary services to the community. In such a situation, business models that focus on protecting the lives of local people, such as that of Adachi, are indispensable for shrinking communities. There are a large number of mountainous areas similar to Hino and Kofu towns across Japan. It is necessary to develop a sustainable method of providing effective support for older people. FDs were initially identified as a form of exclusion of the vulnerable from the society. The Adachi business model resonates with measures that address FDs because it is intended to provide comprehensive protection for the lives of local residents. The business model provides important suggestions for tackling FDs.

Adachi transferred some of his business to his successor (a former colleague) in 2017 when Adachi was 72 years old. The successor established his own company and started operating mobile vending vehicles and stores in Kofu Town. Although Adachi still manages some other vehicles and stores, his business model will be inherited by this successor in near future. Recently, Aikyo has attracted the attention of mobile vending vehicle service operators (business managers and municipal officers) in remote rural areas. These people often visit Adachi Company and learn to manage 'welfare businesses' as a countermeasure to FDs.

Because of the COVID-19 pandemic, many elderly people have remained indoors since April 2020 when the government declared a state of emergency. Therefore, Aikyo's mobile vending vehicle sales are increasing. However, the total sales are still insufficient to offer mobile vending vehicle services without local government subsidies. Under the new restrictions, such as the requirement to maintain social distancing (the so-called 'new normal'), these mobile vending vehicle services may be more important than ever for older residents with disabilities and for people who dislike face-to-face contact with others.

7.2.5   [NB] a Personalized Delivery Shopping Service Business Expanding Across Urban Areas of Japan: Family Network Systems Co., Ltd. (Osaka City, Osaka)

Recently, there has been an increase in the number of startup delivery businesses that incorporate personalized services, mainly in the convenience store industry. These businesses aim to provide support to those who have limited means of shopping and to stimulate demand for such support. On the other hand, most of such businesses are in a tight financial situation. Their challenges include high cost for HR, deliveries, and advertising. This section examines the business of Family Network Systems Co., Ltd. (hereafter referred to as Onemile[4]). The company has operated for approximately 30 years in urban areas with large aging populations. It has met the demand from this aging population by providing personalized delivery shopping services. This section particularly focuses on conditions that enable a business to profit from personalized delivery shopping services in an urban area.

Table 7.9 History of Onemile

Year	Main events
1988	Hotta's Delivery Service starts its operations
1999	Family Network Systems, the first franchise headquarters of a delivery business in Japan, is founded
2005	The Onemile System is introduced, and the comprehensive delivery service business commences
2008	Centralized distribution centres are set up
2009	Ready-to-eat projects are introduced with the help of chefs, and a delivery business of frozen ready-to-eat products to seniors commences
2011	Sales of ready-to-eat products developed with nationally registered dietitians commence
2012	The headquarters of a kitchen studio is completed and a customer call centre is set up
2013	TV shopping services commence, and delivery to all areas of Japan through a partnership with Yamoto Transport commences
2016	A general community support system for delivery of healthy ready-to-eat meals is established
2017	Online shopping using major online shopping sites begins
2018	Online shopping at famous department and convenience stores begins
2020	Rapid increase in sales during the COVID-19 pandemic

Source Family systems' HP and interview survey

Onemile is headquartered in Nishiyodogawa Ward, Osaka City. In 2020, Onemile operated a personalized delivery shopping service business from 75 offices (franchises) in 14 prefectures across Japan. The company is committed to contributing to the community by improving the shopping experience of consumers who consider that they have limited access to shops. Onemile's CEO, Mr. Shigeru Hotta, started the business in 1988 as *Takuhai Senmonten Hotta* (Hotta's Delivery Services) in Nishiyodogawa (Table 7.9). Hotta started his business in a garage of approximately 10 m^2 on the first floor of a built-for-sale house by utilizing his experience of working in a liquor shop since he was a junior high school student. At that time, he sold rice wine and rice that he purchased from Niigata (Hotta 2015). In addition, Onemile started online shopping in 2013. Onemile's online market is expanding rapidly.

In this personalized delivery shopping service, users receive a grocery catalogue[5] every week when a delivery person visits their homes. Users hand a completed order form to the delivery person who comes to deliver the order of the previous week. The business does not charge users membership or delivery fees. There is no minimum number of items for delivery. The person responsible for delivery, who is referred to as a 'supporter', visits the user's home on the same day and the same time every week. Supporters work one of three shifts: morning, afternoon, and evening. They aim to visit five homes in an hour and spend five minutes at each home. They provide personalized delivery services to approximately 45 households per day. An interview survey found that approximately 80% of users place an order on each visit. When a supporter receives an order, they enter data into the

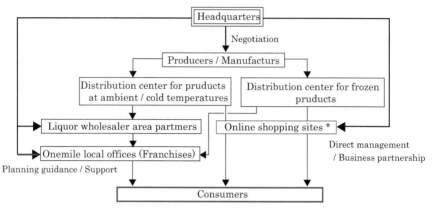

* A company homepage, major online shopping sites,
Department stores' homepages, etc.

Fig. 7.2 Onemile's distribution system. *Source* Based on documents from Family Network Systems
Co., Ltd

Onemile System,[6] the company's own order management system. The entered data
are sent to food producers/manufacturers, distribution centres, and area partners,
where products will be prepared and shipped based on the data. Orders are delivered through different distribution channels depending on their temperature. Items
stored at normal or cold temperatures are sent from producers and manufacturers to
a distribution centre in Kobe City. Frozen products are sent to one in Higashiosaka
City (Fig. 7.2). Products sent to the distribution centre for room temperature products are then delivered to local offices via area partners, which are liquor wholesalers
in 15 areas across Japan. Onemile has partnered with wholesalers working exclu-
sively with Asahi Group Holdings. Onemile has reduced distribution costs by using
existing distribution channels for liquor products. This system allows products to be
delivered to the local office one day before they are delivered to the user. Therefore,
no products are wasted, and the local office does not have excess stock (this system
is referred to as the inventory-free sales system).

Onemile started its online shopping service in 2013 using its skills in product
development and its distribution networks, which it has cultivated since 1988 through
its delivery business. At the beginning, Onemile sold its products only on their homepage. However, since 2017, major online shopping sites such as Amazon, Rakuten
(Japanese major online shopping site), famous department stores and convenience
stores have started selling Onemile's products. Following the expansion of its distribution channels, new customers such as dual-income families and householders with
children started using Onemile's deliveries of frozen ready-to-eat products. Its products are basically a set menu of one main dish and two side dishes, which is a traditional Japanese meal. Japanese-style meals are also popular among wealthy and busy

foreign householders (especially Chinese) who prefer healthy and high quality ready-to-eat products. Therefore, Onemile has a plan to expand its distribution channels to foreign markets (such as Hong Kong and Beijing) in earnest.

Onemile delivers over 1,000 products, mainly groceries such as rice, liquor, and ready-to-eat products as well as various everyday products. The company proposes 10–15 new products weekly. The majority of products in its grocery catalogue are ready-to-eat products of local specialties as well as frozen ready-to-eat products of the company's home brand, Happy Health Dinner (*Kenko Dinner*). Onemile only delivers local products endorsed by Hotta for their taste and quality. Additionally, since 2009, the company has received instructions from external specialists such as chefs, dietitians, and doctors to deliver frozen ready-to-eat products prepared using vacuum processing (Table 7.9). The company develops food products that contribute to older people's health (Photo 7.12). It uses seasonal ingredients, does not add preservatives to products, and maintains the products' optimal nutritional balance while reducing their salt and energy content. All products of the Happy Health Dinner series are handmade. They are sold in sets[7] consisting of main dishes, side dishes, rice, and soup. Users can have different combinations for dinner every day. The dinner series is designed in such a way that it continues to offer new consumer experiences. In

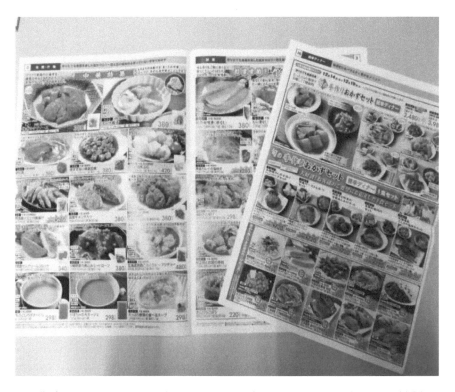

Photo 7.12   A grocery product catalogue developed by Onemile headquarters. Happy Health Dinner on the right (2015, taken by Sasaki)

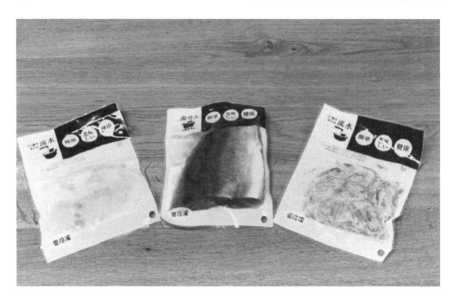

Photo 7.13 Each dish is frozen and packed individually. Cooking methods and use-by dates are displayed (2020, taken by Yamawaki)

addition, each dinner item is individually packed and frozen, so that the characteristics of the ingredients are maintained. They can be stored for a long period of up to six months (Photo 7.13). Onemile's healthy ready-to-eat products and its easy ordering and delivery systems for elderly people are highly regarded by Japanese governments. In 2016, Onemile was designated a 'local medical care industry company'[8] by the Ministry of Economy, Trade and Industry. In addition, Onemile contributes to the revitalization of local food industries (the development of the 'sixth industry'[9]). Specifically, Onemile co-operates with about 20 local governments and develops new menus using their regional fresh foods. For example, Onemile received an offer from Iwami City, which is historically agricultural area that does not have a local speciality, and created a new menu item called a 'bite-sized Iwami pork cutlet'. Iwami pork is fattened by local farmers and cooked by a local food processing company. Onemile sells these meals through its nationwide distribution system.

Approximately 18,000 households use the personalized shopping delivery service (delivery by partners) every month; approximately 80% of the householders are older adults. In contrast, approximately 20,000 households use the online services monthly and many are from the younger generation. In total, about 40% of customers in 2020 are younger people aged less than 34 years old, 30% are middle aged at between 35–64 years old, and about 30% are older adults aged over 65 years old. Moreover, an interview survey of 51 households found that 70.6% of respondents were single-person households and the remainder were married couples. The survey also found that older adult users of Onemile have relatively high incomes (savings) and are healthy. However, 60–75% of them do not own a car. Few older people use government-funded nursing care services. The mean frequency of using Onemile's services is 2.1 times a month. The mean cost of an order is high at approximately 5,200 yen. The company has achieved positive results with a year-on-year growth of over 10% (2015 financial year). It is noteworthy that 90% of Happy Life Dinner customers are returning users. The dinner series is recognized for its health consciousness, long shelf life, and convenience. Onemile asks day service providers to assist with the distribution of advertisements and pamphlets. The company has also gained new customers through various forms of media such as newspapers, radio, TV, and the Internet.

Since April 2020, when the government declared a state of emergency for the COVID-19 pandemic, the demand for ready-to-eat meals has increased rapidly in Japan. The total sales of Onemile's products increased by almost 2.5 times compared with the previous year. With the new requirements, such as social distancing (the so-called 'new normal'), it is expected that the market for healthy online ready-to-eat home meal delivery services may increase further in a post-COVID-19 world.

Given the above, the profitability of Onemile, which operates in urban areas and has many competitors, can be attributed to two factors: cost reduction through an effective distribution system and the development of a wide range of products that meet the expectations of potential customers.

The first factor consists of eliminating food waste and the inventory-free sales strategy through an effective procurement process. Food waste is an issue inherent in any food sales business because food products have shelf lives. However, Onemile does not generate food waste because it only places orders for products ordered by customers. Furthermore, staff from headquarters visit production areas and procure ingredients directly from the source. The company reduces costs through the unified manufacturing and shipping of products. Another advantage of this system is that local offices do not have to keep stock on site because products are delivered directly to them. Moreover, the company reduces distribution costs by using a network of liquor wholesalers. Area partners across the country are distribution hubs; therefore, the local offices of Onemile are located in proximity to area partners. The efficiency of distribution is improved in this way.[10] In addition, it should be noted that Onemile has signed local office contracts with businesses that have already established a solid foundation and have a deep knowledge of the local community. Such businesses include local liquor shops, news agencies, and milk dealers. However, liquor sales licensing has been deregulated. Since deregulation, the number of area partners decreased from 35 to 15. Given this reduction, Onemile cancelled its franchise system[11] and started a new local partnership system in January 2016. Additionally, the company is planning to incorporate a smartphone application for shopping support that is used by over 150 municipal governments. The company is aiming to build a system whereby local partners can ship products ordered on the app. In addition, Onemile's effective distribution network is also useful for the development of online shopping services throughout the entire nation. The headquarters will continue to develop healthy products to meet demand from consumers as well as improve their function as a supplier of such products.

In terms of the second factor, Onemile offers products of local specialties while developing food products with good taste, high quality, and balanced nutrition that can be stored for a long period of time. The company's original Happy Health Dinner series have proven particularly popular with an increasing number of consumers. The amount spent on these products by each customer is high because they are sold in sets. Currently, various welfare businesses, not only those focused on helping people with limited access to shops, are increasingly interested in providing services to older people suffering from undernutrition and receiving government-funded nursing care services. In contrast, Hotta considers that it is more important to prevent undernutrition and the need for nursing care among older adults. He also points out that to achieve this, it is necessary to build a system for the provision of meals with balanced nutrition to healthy older people. Moreover, he believes this model would make a profitable business. Hotta considers that there is further potential demand for Onemile's services from healthy older adults because Onemile provides food products to help them maintain their health. It is a new style of business.

Onemile has expanded its services. It is currently providing paid services in the following areas: purchasing services on behalf of users, home maintenance services (such as putting garbage out and changing light bulbs), and safety watch services. Older people are concentrated in urban areas, and many live alone or with a partner. The importance of everyday support services has been increasingly recognized in the community because of this social situation, which is a growing trend.

7.2.6 [NB] Travel for Elderly People on a Free Shopping Bus Service: Kurukuru Bus (Fukushima City, Fukushima Prefecture)

One of the measures to address the FD issue is shopping buses. Although they are not legally defined as 'shopping buses', the term is used to describe a bus for passengers who want to shop. In general, such services provide a means of transport to a shopping destination for residents in areas without retail shops nearby and where public transport is inconvenient.

In recent years, Demand Responsive Transport (DRT)—not only for shopping but also for visiting hospitals and public facilities—has become widespread. With the revision of the Road Transportation Law in 2006, DRT has been introduced in many areas, mainly in rural areas. However, to introduce DRT, it is necessary to co-ordinate with existing public transport and taxi operators in local public transportation conventions, so it is not easy to introduce DRT in urban areas. Commercial facilities included in the shopping bus service route can be broadly classified into two: commercial districts such as central shopping districts and one specific commercial facility. The former facilities are often operated mainly by the Chamber of Commerce and Industry as a measure to revitalize the central shopping street. The latter is often operated by a commercial facility to attract customers.

Most shopping buses charge fares, except when they operate in large commercial facilities. However, shopping bus fares are cheap compared with those of local buses

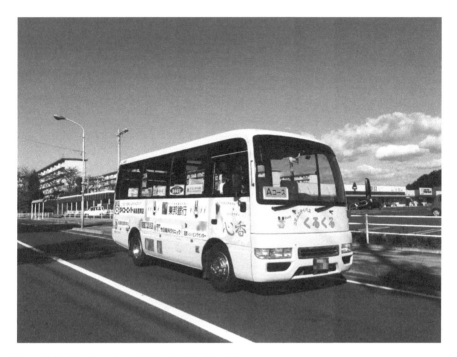

Photo 7.14 Kurukuru bus (2015, taken by Tanaka)

and taxis, and many rides cost only 100–200 yen. In addition, there are cases where the fare is discounted for shopping at the target commercial facility. These bus fares are an important source of revenue for maintaining the operations of most shopping buses.

However, the 'Kurukuru Bus', a shopping bus that operates within the Horai housing complex in Fukushima city, Fukushima prefecture, is free (Photo 7.14). 'Kurukuru' is a mimetic word meaning 'circulation' in English. The bus is operated by an NPO to improve the environment of the housing complex. Operating costs are covered by the accumulation of original efforts and ingenuity, including donations from major users and commercial facilities. Below, we explain the operation, the introduction process, and the system for maintaining the operation.

The Horai housing complex is located on a low mountain about 7 km from the central part of Fukushima city (Fig. 7.3). This housing complex was developed in the early 1970s and consists of many detached houses and some apartment buildings. The initial planned population was 15,100 and the area is 225.1 ha. By 2004, a total of 4,096 houses had been constructed.

In November 2015, the population of Horai district, including the housing complex, was 11,715. Because the housing complex is in the mountains, there are many slopes that are difficult for elderly people to climb. The Horai Shopping Centre (Horai SC), which has a local capital supermarket as its core shop, is located in the centre of the housing complex. There are home centres and specialty shops on the

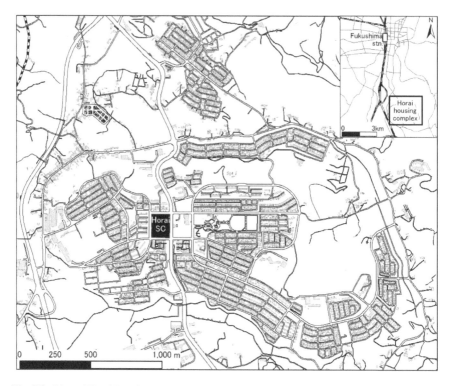

Fig. 7.3 Map of Horai housing complex in 2015. *Source* Iwama ed. (2017)

same site (Photo 7.15). In addition, city-related branch offices, post offices, banks, and other facilities are concentrated on the next block. The residents of the housing complex can maintain a comfortable life as long as they can come to this area.

The Kurukuru Bus starts from and terminates at Horai SC. The housing complex is almost covered by three circulation routes that take about 20–25 min per round. A bus with a capacity of 29 people runs every day except Sunday from 9 a.m. to around 4 p.m.; there are five services a day for each route. Bus stops are installed at intervals of several hundred metres. However, the service operates flexibly for the convenience of users, such as stopping for passengers who want to board even at places without bus stops (Photo 7.16).

The Kurukuru Bus (represented by Ms. Etsuko Kobayashi) was started in 2008 by the Horai Machizukuri Zeene voluntary organization. 'Machizukuri' means 'community development' in English and 'Zeene' means 'nice' in the dialect around Fukushima city. The Kurukuru Bus service was triggered by the dissolution of the public corporation for local housing that developed and maintained the Horai housing complex and operated the Horai SC. Previously, Horai SC had been operated by a public corporation, but responsibility was shifted to a private company following its dissolution. To maintain sales that could be managed by private capital shops within the SC and to provide transportation for residents unable to drive cars, a shopping

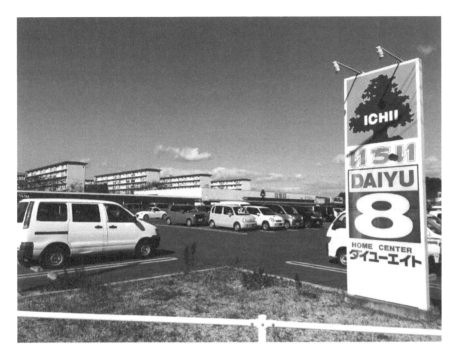

Photo 7.15 Horai shopping center (2015, taken by Tanaka)

bus service was started. The voluntary organization acquired the legal status of NPO in 2013 and became the Machizukuri Zeene Corporation NPO.

Since its establishment, the corporation has had an office in a part of the specialty shopping district of Horai SC. The office is open to passengers and is a haven for those who finish shopping and are waiting for the bus to depart. Water and tea are provided there, and people waiting for the bus sit on the sofa and chat.

Since the start of operations in June 2008, there have been around 15,000–18,000 passengers per year, with an average of 60–80 passengers a day. Considering that most passengers take round trips, there are between 30 and 40 regular passengers per day. However, the number of passengers varies depending on the day, such as on the regular supermarket sales days where the number of passengers is extremely high. A typical pattern for passengers is to come to Horai SC on a bus at around 10 a.m. and return on one that leaves Horai SC in the afternoon. In this case, the user can stay at the SC for about an hour and can complete business at a facility such as a city office branch or bank as well as go shopping. In the supermarket, there will also be announcements that inform passengers that the bus is about to depart. If passengers finish shopping early, they can relax and wait for the bus at the meeting place in the office.

In addition, the Kurukuru Bus is not only for SC users but also for many users of the adjacent Fukushima City Hall Horai Learning Centre. Various events are held at the centre, which is attached to the city office branch, and it is used for club activities. For this reason, some residents participate in such events using the Kurukuru Bus.

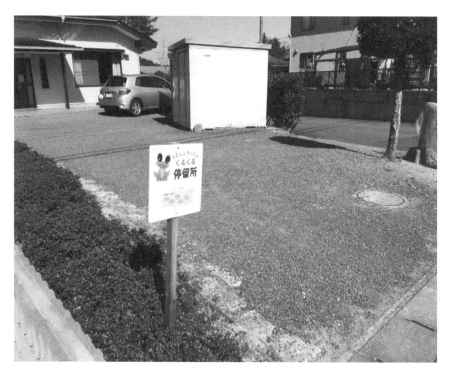

Photo 7.16 Bus stop of Kurukuru bus (2015, taken by Tanaka)

In this way, the Kurukuru Bus has a certain number of passengers, but it has been difficult to secure operating funds. The main expenditures are bus leasing costs, including driver labour and fuel. The operating funds are derived from various sources, and the following are some major examples. The first is the Kurukuru Bus paid membership system, supported by residents (including bus users) in the Horai housing complex who understand the significance of the service. Members pay 1,000 yen each month to Zeene. Some supporters become paid members even though they do not normally use the bus.

The second source of revenue is sales of advertising space on buses. Advertising fees have been obtained from about 15 organizations, such as shops and banks in the SC, for painting the exterior of the Kurukuru Bus and attaching advertisements to its windows. Third, Zeene has earned income from power sales through solar power generation, which is part of the environmental town development. Electricity is sold by installing solar panels on the roofs of offices and on the grounds outside the housing complex with the assistance of the national and prefectural governments. There are also donations from organizations and volunteers that support the Kurukuru Bus initiative. Operating expenses have been covered by these initiatives.

In the discussion of counter-measures against FDs, some believe that home delivery is the best solution. The author agrees that this would ensure a stable food supply. However, home delivery is not the optimal measure for maintaining a rich diet and health. To maintain the health of the elderly, it i s essential for them to go out as well as to eat properly. They can maintain their physical health by walking and maintain their intellectual activity by interacting with people. Going out is indispensable in preventing dementia and avoiding the need for care, and shopping can be said to provide an appropriate form of exercise. When one speaks to them, one can see their thought processes. They are thinking about the menu for the next few days. They use a supermarket flyer to determine which ingredients are affordable and base their purchase decisions according to the ingredients left at home. They choose what to buy by observing what is available at the shop. They do not forget to bring their bags and gain reward points. In this way, they are going shopping while remaining mentally active.

When the author got on the Kurukuru Bus, it had at most 10 passengers. The driver and passengers conversed when getting on and off the bus and the passengers talked during the journey. The conversation began with the weather and expanded to sales at the SC shop, point cards, and ways to cook the ingredients bought at the shop. The inside of the bus becomes a salon, and the connections between them are fostered through common shopping topics. This is a tremendous by-product of the shopping bus's use, which is superior to convenient home delivery and solitary visits by car.

Many elderly people can drive their own cars and actively engage in social activities. For such people, obtaining food is a trivial matter. However, many elderly people do not like social activities and remain in their homes. Aged housebound people tend to be less intelligent and physically active and have a higher risk of requiring care and suffering dementia. However, they cannot live without buying groceries. In other words, food shopping is an essential opportunity to go out. A shopping bus is an effective opportunity for aged housebound people to communicate with others.

In Japan, the significance of buses is often talked about only in terms of income and expenditure, but the health and human connection of residents traveling by bus are an invisible form of regional revenue. The shopping bus can be said to be an intermediate good that produces it.

7.2.7 [NB]a New Business Type: Co-operation Between a Local Shopping Centre, Local People, and a Transfer and Support Company to Create a Sustainable Community Space for Elderly People (Izumisano City, Osaka Prefecture)

This is a new type of business to support the elderly by creating sustainable and free community spaces with convenient transport. A local shopping centre (Icora Mall Izumisano[12]), local people (Fureai Centre & Salon[13]), and a transfer and support company (Fukushi Life[14]) co-manage this business in Izumisano City, Osaka Prefecture. The unique aspects of this business are (1) The S.C. pays almost all the expenses of this community space and provides a free bus, and (2) it offers a paid welfare transport service for elderly people who need care or support. This business started in July 2017.

Fureai Centre & Salon is managed by local volunteers and has free community spaces for local (mainly elderly) people. The salon is located in Icora Mall Izumisano, a local shopping centre in Izumisano City (Photo 7.17). Fureai Centre & Salon has six areas, each with about 30 m^2 of floor space. The areas include a volunteer's office, an exercise space, a karaoke space, a mah-jong space, and a rest space. Local clubs such as sports clubs and a cultural school can use these spaces freely with an advance reservation (Photo 7.18). The members of these clubs can enjoy shopping in the shopping centre either before or after their club activities. Generally, local sports and cultural clubs use public facilities such as gymnastics halls and lecture halls established by social welfare councils. However, in 2017, the social welfare councils in Izumisano City moved to suburban areas, where it is difficult for carless elderly people to visit. Therefore, many elderly people visit Fureai Centre & Salon for their leisure activities. Approximately 500 people a week visit Fureai Centre & Salon (June 2020). Because of this salon, patronage of Icora Mall Izumisano is increasing.

Many elderly members are content to drive private cars or use public transportation to the shopping centre. However, carless people in areas of poor public transportation

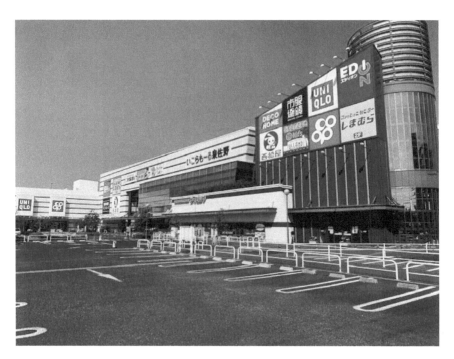

Photo 7.17 Icora Mall Izumisano (2020, taken by Noguchi)

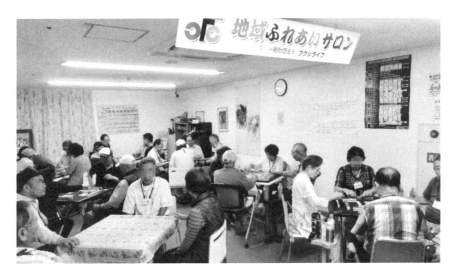

Photo 7.18 Fureai Centre & Salon (2019, taken by Noguchi)

seldom visit Icora Mall Izumisano independently. Therefore, the salon offers the 'Fureai Centre & Salon' free transportation service for these people (for members only; this service is offered in poor food access areas). 6,472 people used this free transportation service during April 2019–May 2020 (Fig. 7.4) (Photo 7.19).[15] In addition, for people with limited ability to support themselves, Fureai Centre &

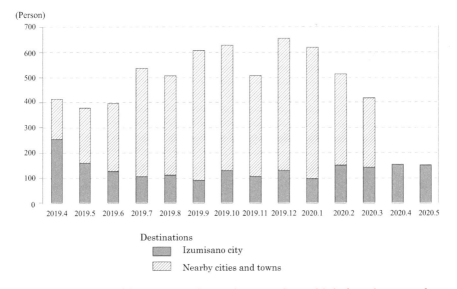

Fig. 7.4 The number of free transportation service users. *Source* Made from documents from Fukushi Life

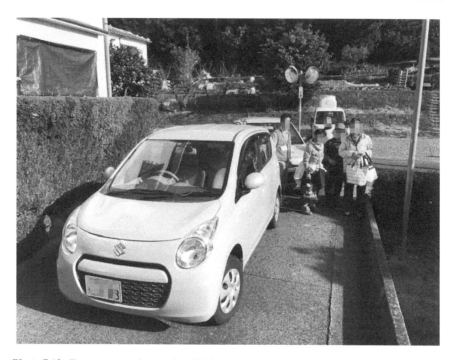

Photo 7.19 Free transportation service (2019, taken by Noguchi)

Salon offers paid welfare transportation. The service is not free but is covered by elder care insurance. The number of peoples who used the paid welfare transportation service during the same period is 22 (Photo 7.20).

Many running costs of these services are paid by Icora Mall Izumisano. For example, the rent for Fureai Centre & Salon is free. Furniture, including tables, chairs, and partitions, is also offered by the shopping centre. The utility bills of this salon are also covered by Icora Mall Izumisano, as are the running costs of the free bus. This is how Fureai Centre & Salon can maintain its activities.

Icora Mall Izumisano, which opened in 2000, is a local shopping centre located about two kilometres from Izumisano train station. It has a floor space of 33,805 m^2 with a food supermarket and many tenanted shops, including clothing stores, volume-sales electronics retailers, restaurants, and a branch office of an entertainment agency. This shopping centre is popular, but it has recently encountered strong competition from Rinku Premium Outlet, which is one of the largest outlet malls in Japan. This outlet mall has 49,600 m^2 of floor space in 2020 and attracts many customers from large areas beyond Izumisano City. In the face of this competition, Icora Mall Izumisano started Fureai Centre & Salon and transport services to attract local elderly people, especially disadvantaged shoppers.

Mr. Noguchi Hidetoshi (CEO of Fukushi Life), Mr. Nakako Yasumitsu (Operation Manager of Icora Mall Izumisano) and Mr. Asano Masaya (CEO of Tokyo Rope MFG Co., Ltd) developed this business. Fukushi Life is a general incorporated association

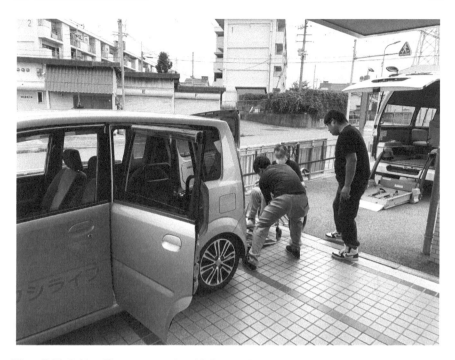

Photo 7.20   Paid welfare transportation (2019, taken by Noguchi)

that runs a nursery, nursing home, and a temporary training school for paid welfare transportation vehicle drivers. The paid welfare transportation is a kind of volunteer taxi service with private vehicles. Generally, only professional drivers with class 2 licences can drive or chauffeur commercial passenger vehicles such as buses, taxis, and limousines. However, the Japanese government permits some kinds of volunteer taxi passenger transport in private vehicles in some areas (for more detail, please see Chapter 7, Sect. 7.2.7). The paid welfare transportation service is one such service. It provides a special door-to-door transport service for members such as elderly and disabled people. Health and welfare certificate holders (i.e. care workers) are permitted to drive paid welfare transportation vehicles, even without a class 2 driving licence. Paid welfare transportation includes the following services: (1) transporting users to their destinations, (2) assisting passengers to board and alight, and (3) providing support while the passengers are shopping or undergoing medical examinations.

Mr. Noguchi has been engaged in welfare services for the elderly for a long time, and he is strongly aware of two facts. (1) Leisure activities, such as participating in the local community, cultural and sports clubs, as well as shopping, are necessary for elderly people. However, many elderly people have difficulty going out owing to a lack of transportation. In addition, many older elderly persons over the age of 75 years have difficulty going out without physical support. We should consider suitable ways to facilitate going out for house-bound elderly people. If familiar care workers accompany them, they can enjoy leisure activities with an easy mind. (2) Care work is important for countries with ageing populations such as Japan. However, because of the lack of long-term financial resources from care insurance, care worker salaries in nursing homes are too low.[16] This is a major reason for the dearth of care workers in Japan. We should create a new system to increase the incomes of care workers.

To help solve these problems, above three key persons developed this business. If many elderly people use Fureai Centre & Salon, they can enjoy their leisure activities there and Icora Mall Izumisano will attract new customers. In addition, if elderly people use the paid welfare transportation vehicles driven by familiar care workers, care workers will receive additional income. It is safe to say that Fureai Centre & Salon has already achieved results. On the other hand, many people do not use paid welfare transportation vehicles to reach Fureai Centre & Salon. The service is less convenient now, because there are fewer of these vehicles than buses and taxis. Therefore, Mr. Noguchi plans to establish a new online paid welfare bus allocation control system similar to that of Uber.

7.3 The Possibility of Volunteer Taxi Passenger Transportation by Private Vehicle

Volunteer taxi passenger transportation by private vehicles is expected to play an important role in public transport in poor food access areas. Generally, volunteer taxi services are managed by NPOs with so-called 'white number plate cars' (in Japan, professional transport vehicles such as taxis and buses use green or black plates). The governing bodies are usually not automobile transport businesses. Volunteer taxi services already operate in some areas of Japan. However, currently, to maintain a balance with automobile transport companies, volunteer taxi passenger transport is restricted to many points, including scope of operations and contents of activities. However, at the National Strategic Special Zone Advisory Council in October 2015, the Prime Minister of Japan announced his intent to deregulate volunteer taxi passenger transportation. Therefore, such activities will be expanded in the future.[17]

We will discuss the introduction of volunteer taxi passenger transportation systems in Japan and introduce some case studies of depopulated communities' volunteer taxi passenger transportation.

7.3.1 The Expansion of Areas with Poor Public Transportation and Volunteer Taxi Passenger Transportation

Since the 1970s, when so-called 'motorization' progressed rapidly, the number of public transport users has decreased. In addition, owing to changes in subsidies for fixed-route buses and the deregulation of bus businesses, it has become more difficult to maintain their operations in regional and rural areas. Therefore, many bus companies have withdrawn from or shortened their bus routes from less populated areas (Tanaka 2009). In poor transportation areas, many people without private cars or who cannot drive have difficulty in maintaining a minimal living environment, including access to nearby grocery shops or medical institutions.

To improve these living environments, new transportation systems were started and expanded in the 2000s. These new systems reflect out-of-the-box thinking. These transportation systems, represented by DRT, can be operated flexibly according to local needs. These systems are useful in covering poorly populated towns and villages where houses are scattered. The need for these new forms of transport continues to increase. Therefore, the Japanese government has made an exception to normal practice by permitting commercial transport by cars with white number plates, which is a kind of volunteer taxi passenger transport service operated by NPOs. The number of such exceptions is increasing. In this situation, the government revised the Road Transportation Law in October 2006. This revision provided a legal basis for white-plate car transport and it became easier to operate such systems legally.

7.3.2 The History and Outline of Volunteer Taxi Passenger Transportation

Volunteer taxi passenger transportation by private vehicles can be classified into 'municipal government volunteer taxi transportation', 'volunteer taxi transportation in depopulated communities', and 'welfare non-fee transportation' (Table 7.10).[18] To start a volunteer taxi transportation system, a management committee must be established. The management committees are composed of representatives from the local government, local transportation bureaus, local residents, NPOs, transportation companies, and other parties. This meeting should discuss: (1) the necessity for volunteer taxi transportation, (2) the scope of activities for these services, and (3) the fees charged to customers. With the approval of the management committee, the volunteer taxi passenger transportation system is registered with the Ministry of Land, Infrastructure and Transport (usually deputized by the assistant director of the transportation bureaus) (Ministry of Land, Infrastructure and Transport 2015). The conditions for registration are: (1) a lack of bus and taxi companies that creates a need for alternative transportation, and local residents, municipalities, and local transportation companies agree to establish a volunteer taxi service in the area. (2) Sufficient

Table 7.10 Classification of volunteer taxi transportation

Classification		Outline
Municipal government volunteer taxi transportation	Transportatioin blank areas	This service is only offered to residents in transportation blank areas. This transportation is managed by the municipal government
	Municipal welfare transport	This service is only offered to physically disabled people who have difficulty moving by themselves or using public transport. This transport is managed by the municipal government. Users must resister for membership. Basically, this is individual transport (door to door)
Volunteer taxi transportation in depopulated communities		This service is only offered to residents in transportation blank areas and their relatives. This transport is managed by an NPO or other organization. Users must be members of the operating body
Welfare no-fee transportation		This service is only offered to physically disabled people who have difficulty in moving by themselves or using public transport. This transport is managed by an NPO or other organization. It uses wagons with a capacity of fewer than 11 people. Basically, this is individual transport (door to door)

Source Ministry of Land, Infrastructure and Transport, Road Transport Bureau, Passenger Transport Division (2015)

safety measures (such as a management system, skilled drivers, maintenance systems, and an emergency contact system) have been adopted.

The municipal government's volunteer taxi transportation is managed by local governments. In contrast, a depopulated community's volunteer taxi transportation and welfare non-fee transportation are operated by NPOs or other organizations, and users of these services must register in advance. Welfare non-fee transportation services are only offered to physically disabled people who have difficulty in moving by themselves or using public transport. However, a depopulated community's volunteer taxi transportation service is offered to every resident including healthy people living in poor access areas.

7.3.3   Examples of Volunteer Taxi Practices in Depopulated Communities

If local people who meet certain conditions (such as driving experience, age, and private car ownership) register as drivers, they may provide the operating body with drivers and vehicles. In short, it is not really necessary for the operating body to purchase its own cars or hire drivers. It can save initial costs.[19] This is one of the greatest advantages of volunteer taxi transportation. It is safe to say that volunteer taxi transportation makes good use of local human resources and property to provide transport for residents in poor access areas. Volunteer taxi transportation is a bargaining chip for maintaining transportation systems in depopulated areas.

The first trial of volunteer taxi transportation began in Kamikatsu town, Tokushima prefecture, in 2003. This town is located in a mountainous area and has serious problems with depopulation and aging. There is no taxi company and few fixed public bus routes. Therefore, the Japanese government permitted the establishment of volunteer taxi transportation in this town as a pilot program in a special district for structural reform. From this experiment in Kamikatsu town and the revision of the Road Transportation Law in 2006, volunteer taxi transportation systems have penetrated the nation's depopulated communities (Table 7.11).

The typical management method is as follows. First, the operating body acts as a call centre and connects customers with drivers by telephone. For example, if a person wants to use this service to go shopping at a supermarket, the person calls the call centre operators and tells them the pick-up point, destination, and time. Then, the call centre operator offers this order to a driver. If the driver accepts it, the driver goes to the meeting point at the appointed time to collect the passenger. If a driver declines, the operator seeks an alternative driver. Usually, the fare is paid directly to drivers by fare tickets issued by the operating body. Passenger fares should not exceed actual expenses, including fuel and labour costs. In short, the passenger fare must be compensation for the service, which must not be a commercial activity. Generally, a passenger fare is composed of a fixed 'geisha charge' (charge for a car on the way to collect a passenger) and a 'travel fare' determined in proportion to the distance travelled. The basic operating area is limited to the municipality. However, if either point of departure or destination is located in the area where operations are permitted, the vehicle can carry passengers beyond the permitted area. In short, it is possible for users to shop in an adjacent municipality's supermarket using this form of transportation.

Thus, volunteer taxi transportation supports disadvantaged shoppers effectively using local resources, and this is the trump card for transportation in poor food access areas. It is expected that this transportation will expand further through depopulated poor food access areas. This method will become increasingly important in the future.

Table 7.11 Major volunteer taxi transportation services using private cars

Municipal	Operational Body	Operational areas	Use of service beyond the operational area	Fare
Ishikari City, Hoppaido Pref.	Attaka Life Support (NPO)	Atsuta Ward	Not allowed	Distance-based system
Sai Village, Aomori Pref.	Sai Village Council of Social Welfare	Sai Village	Permitted (if taxi starts from or arrives at operational area)	Zonal tariff system
Kitakami City, Iwate Pref.	Kuchinai (NPO)	Kunai District, Kitakami City	Not allowed	Distance-based system
Hitachiota City, Ibaraki Pref.	Hitachiota City Satomi Chamber of Commerce and Industry	Satomi District, Hitachiota City	Permitted (if taxi starts from or arrives at operational area)	Distance-based toll
Goka Town, Ibaraki Pref.	Goka Town Council of Social Welfare	Goka Town	Permitted (if taxi starts from or arrives at operational area)	Time charge system + fuel expenses
Kiryu City and Midori City, Gumma Pref.	Group 28 (NPO)	Kurohone District, Kiryu City, and Azuma District, Midorino City	Permitted (if taxi starts from or arrives at operational area)	Distance-based system
Minamiboso City, Chiba Pref.	Minamiboso City Council of Social Welfare	Minamiboso City	Within Minamiboso City, Tateyama City, Mamogawa City, and Kyonan Town	Time charge system + distance-based system
Hida City, Gifu Pref.	Kitahida Chamber of Commerce and Industry	Kawai District and Miyakawa District, Hida City	Not allowed	100 yen
Toyone Village, Aichi Pref.	Toyone Village Silber Human Resources center	Toyone Village	Permitted (if taxi starts from or arrives at operational area)	Zonal tariff system
Mima City, Tokushima Pref.	Koyadaira (NPO)	Kiyadaira District, Mima City	Permitted (if taxi starts from or arrives at operational area)	Distance-based system
Kamikatsu Village, Tokushima Pref.	Zero Waste Academy (NPO)	Kamikatsu Village	Permitted (if taxi starts from or arrives at operational area)	Distance-based system
Ino Town, Kochi Pref.	Ino Town Council of Social Welfare	Inomachi Motokawa District, Ino Town	Permitted (if taxi starts from or arrives at operational area)	Distance-based system

(continued)

Table 7.11 (continued)

Municipal	Operational Body	Operational areas	Use of service beyond the operational area	Fare
Yusuhara Town, Kochi Pref.	Kizuna (NPO)	Hatsuse District and Matsubara District, Yusuhara Town	Permitted (if taxi starts from or arrives at operational area)	Zonal tariff system

Notes

1. We collected information by Ministry of Agriculture, Forestry and Fisheries (2011), Ministry of Economy, Trade and Industry (2015), and Ministry of Economy, Trade and Industry (2011).
2. Some counter-measures apply only to certain issues.
3. In our interview survey, many older women answered as follows: 'I do lots of housekeeping every day for family members. Housekeeping is very heavy and unskilled labour, but few people appreciate our endless housekeeping work. On the other hand, Nakayoshi's work is heavy, but creative. We have the gratification of knowing that we contribute to local society using our housekeeping skills. And many people appreciate our volunteer work. Moreover, we can get fulfilment by working toward a goal with people of different generations. That is why we find Nakayoshi's volunteer work attractive.'
4. Onemile is the delivery department of Family Network Systems Co., Ltd.
5. Local specialties and ready-to-eat products made by Onemile are shown in full colour in over 1 6 pages of the weekly grocery catalogue.
6. This is the original ordering system developed with Itochu Corporation in 2005.
7. A side-dish subscription set includes a main dish and two side dishes for 3,480 yen for five meals. A full subscription set includes side dish sets, rice, and soup for 3,980 yen for five meals.
8. The Ministry of Economy, Trade and Industry promotes a medical care industry policy. This policy aims to increase life expectancy and create new industries. If the government increases the number of elderly people who live heathy lives, it will not only improve quality of life but also save money on social security benefits. https://www.meti.go.jp/policy/mono_info_service/healthcare/01metihealthcarepolicy.pdf. Accessed 14 August 2020.
9. In a bid to create new regional jobs, the Japanese government has paid attention to the presence of abundant primary industry products (especially regional fresh foods) and proposed a 'food processing and distribution complex initiative' to combine the primary, secondary and tertiary industries into a sixth industry to generate new added value for the region.
10. The population of the local commercial area of each local office is determined by local authorities.

11. Onemile no longer requires area partners to pay for membership, education, training, or royalties.
12. The shopping centre is owned by Tokyo Rope MFG Co., Ltd.
13. Their real estate is managed by Xymax Kansai Corporation.
14. http://fukushi-life.jp/.
15. Due to new coronavirus, Fukushi life restricts the operation areas of the free transportation service since 2020.4.
16. The average income in Japan is about 5.52 million yen, while that of care workers is 3.40 million yen (Ministry of Health, Labour and Welfare 2018).
17. The Japanese government authorizes official volunteer taxi transportation under certain conditions, such as operating within a national strategic special zone. The Prime Minister's declaration aimed to promote tourist use of volunteer taxis in rural areas. However, this deregulation also made it possible for residents to use the system.
18. The Japanese government changed the name of this form of public transportation from 'depopulated community volunteer taxi transportation' to 'volunteer taxis as public transportation in blank areas' in 2006. Nevertheless, the former name is widely used.
19. Of course, some operating bodies are prepared for exclusive cars and drivers. This is because they cannot secure a sufficient number of drivers from residents, or they question residents' driving skills.

References

Hotta S (2015) Efforts to make the Onemile personalized delivery shopping service business for aging people. Food industry for tomorrow Nov 21–26 (Japanese)

Iwama N (ed) (2011) Food deserts issues: food deserts and isolated society. Association of Agriculture and Forestry Statistics, Tokyo (Japanese)

Iwama N (ed) (2013) Food deserts issues: revised and updated edition: food deserts and isolated society. Association of Agriculture and Forestry Statistics, Tokyo (Japanese)

Iwama N (ed) (2017) Urban food deserts issues: urban food deserts in low-social capital areas. Association of Agriculture and Forestry Statistics, Tokyo (Japanese)

Ministry of Agriculture, Forestry and Fisheries (2011) Remarkable case studies to resolve the inconveniences and difficulties in food shopping (Japanese). https://www.maff.go.jp/primaff/koho/seminar/2011/attach/pdf/110802_10.pdf. Accessed 14 Aug 2020

Ministry of Economy, Trade and Industry (2011) Support manual for disadvantaged shoppers version 2.0 (Japanese). http://warp.da.ndl.go.jp/info:ndljp/pid/8380059/www.meti.go.jp/policy/economy/distribution/manyuaruver2.pdf. Accessed 14 Aug 2020

Ministry of Economy, Trade and Industry (2015) Support manual for disadvantaged shoppers version 3.0 (Japanese). https://www.meti.go.jp/policy/economy/distribution/150427_manual_2.pdf. Accessed 14 Aug 2020

Ministry of Economy, Trade and Industry (2019) As for support services for disadvantaged shoppers (Japanese). https://www.meti.go.jp/policy/economy/distribution/kaimonojakusyashien.html. Accessed 3 Aug 2020

Ministry of Health, Labour and Welfare (2018) Basic Survey on Wage Structure (Japanese). https://www.mhlw.go.jp/toukei/itiran/roudou/chingin/kouzou/z2018/dl/13.pdf. Accessed 3 Aug 2020

Ministry of Land, Infrastructure and Transport, Road Transport Bureau, Passenger Transport Division (2015) The plactical instruction manual of volunteer taxi passenger transportation. https://wwwtb.mlit.go.jp/kanto/jidou_koutu/tabi2/jikayo/date/jikayo_yuusyo.pdf. Accessed 15 Mar 2021 (Japanese)

NPO Zenkoku-ido Service Network (2015) Information regarding transportation legal system (Japanese). http://www.zenkoku-ido.net/laws.php. Accessed 3 Aug 2020

Sakamoto K (2010) The story of companies friendly to the vulnerable in society. Kindai-Sales Co, Tokyo (Japanese)

Seki M (2015) Assisting disadvantaged shoppers in mountainous areas. Shinhyoron Publishing, Tokyo (Japanese)

Tanaka K (2009) Issues and reviews of public transportation in intermediate and mountainous areas. Association of Economic Geographers 55:33–48 (Japanese)

Yakushiji T (ed) (2015) Food access issues in a super-aging society. Harvest-sha, Inc., Tokyo (Japanese)

About the Book

In our previous book (Iwama 2011), we reported that food deserts (FDs) were poor food access areas[1] (streets where shops are shuttered). However, our current research shows other characteristics of Japanese FDs. Social capital (SC) is an especially important factor. Therefore, in this book,[2] we redefine an FD as a place that satisfies two conditions: (1) many socially vulnerable people (especially elderly people) live there, and (2) the shopping environment has deteriorated (there are fewer nearby grocery shops and decreased food access) and/or local ties with families and neighbours have been diluted (there is decreased mutual assistance and a decline in local SC). Moreover, we estimate that the most serious FDs are located in urban areas. Therefore, we researched the conditions of urban FDs in the central areas of Tokyo, a prefectural governmental city, and a small city. In addition, we introduced notable countermeasures against FDs in several categories. Below are five findings from our research.

The Elderly Population of Urban Areas and the Risk of Isolation from Local Society Have Increased (Chapter 2)

In Chap. 2, we explained the potential for future population ageing and the changes in population structure in urban areas. The older elderly (people aged over 75 years) have generally more difficulty in shopping and cooking than the younger elderly (65–74 years old), and the population of older elderly people will rapidly increase in the near future. This means that the risk of FDs in Japan will increase further.

Elderly households are concentrated in the central areas of big cities. The population structure of Tokyo shows that the proportion of elderly people is higher in the three central Tokyo wards (the Minato, Chuou, and Chiyoda wards). The proportion of single households is also higher in these three wards. The population structure of central Tokyo is diverse. Many high-income white-collar people live there. Moreover,

N. Iwama et al., *Urban Food Deserts in Japan*, International Perspectives in Geography 15, https://doi.org/10.1007/978-981-16-0893-3

there are also high proportions of unemployed people, young people (20–29 years old), and foreign residents in central Tokyo. In short, single elderly residents share their living environments with many different kinds of people. In such a diverse area, it is difficult for residents to build local SC. This fact suggests that elderly people can easily become isolated from local communities in urban areas.

The Dimensions of Social Capital in Food Deserts (Chapter 3)

In Chap. 3, we discussed food access and SC. These are significant living environment factors that impair elderly people's eating habits. The dimension of food access is well-known, and in this book, we introduced some methods to measure it.

In contrast, the dimension of SC is not well recognized. SC refers to social networks (ties with people and groups) and normative consciousness based on trust and reciprocity. If people or groups trust each other, have sufficiently good relationships to help each other, and communicate positively and regularly, they can feel a sense of security. In high-SC areas, even if there are few nearby grocery shops, neighbours and relatives support the carless elderly by shopping on their behalf and sharing daily meals with them. On the other hand, in low-SC areas, elderly people tend to be isolated from society and stay in their houses all day long. In addition, even if there are sufficient nearby grocery shops, the elderly people's eating habits tend to be worse than those in high-SC areas.

The following indices are generally used to measure SC: (1) participation in social organizations with a vertical social structure, (2) participation in social organizations with a horizontal social structure, (3) level of relationships with neighbours, (4) breadth of relationships with neighbours, (5) feelings of trust, and (6) reciprocity norms. However, it is difficult to measure SC using all of the above indices. Recently, scholars in social epidemiology and other academic fields have enthusiastically studied the relationship between people's health and SC. In this book, we introduce two ways to measure SC. However, to universalize SC measurement, further refinement is necessary.

The Conditions of Urban Food Deserts (Chapers 4–6)

In Chaps. 4–6, we analysed elderly people's eating habits and living environments. These studies are summarized below.

Districts A and B in Central Tokyo (Chapter 4)

Minato City is generally considered to be a 'celebrity' area, and such areas are free from forms of social exclusion such as FDs. However, the resident structure is diverse in this area, and the rate of poverty has also increased among the local elderly people. In this book, we discussed the conditions of urban FDs in the case study areas of Districts A and B in Minato City, Tokyo. There are few food access areas in District A. On the other hand, there are many grocery shops in District B and food is relatively accessible. However, many of these groceries are upmarket individual stores and supermarkets that sell exclusive products.

We found that many older residents are at high risk of malnutrition (District A: 44.6%; District B: 55.2%). The common characteristics of elderly people at high risk of malnutrition are relatively low incomes and poor SC. It is safe to say that urban FDs exist in both areas.

Minato City is a high-status residential area, and many self-made high-income people have moved there. On the other hand, because of its high inheritance tax, many elderly residents have left. In addition, some low-income elderly people live in public housing in Minato City. Many low-income people moved there before the 1980s, after which time the land prices in Minato City rose dramatically. Then, they remained there and grew old. The most serious victims of the FD in this area are the low-income elderly people who have no ties with the local community. In addition, some high-income residents also have unhealthy eating habits and a high malnutrition risk. The urban renewal districts of central Tokyo are prosperous areas with many high-rise apartments and upmarket commercial facilities. However, low-class housing, including public housing, still exists in Minato City and social problems such as FD issues prevail there. We must consider central Tokyo in a comprehensive manner.

The Central Area of Prefectural Capital City C (Chapter 5)

In the centre of prefectural governmental City C (about 1 km from the main train station), although a few grocery shops remain, including a department store and a general merchandise shop, many shops have moved from the central shopping street to suburban areas about 1–2 km from the main station, and the outskirts of this city centre are largely comprised of poor food access areas. Our questionnaire survey showed that many city-centre residents go shopping on foot or by bicycle and have no difficulty obtaining daily food. Few residents were interested in healthy dietary habits. Our research on healthy eating habits (the 'investigation of food diversity' score) showed that almost half of the residents were at high risk of malnutrition. These high-risk elderly people mainly live in the city centre around the central shopping streets. We also found these elderly people on the outskirts of the city centre. There are still some grocery shops in the city centre. The shopping environments in the city centre seem adequate. Therefore, the local government does not offer any support services for elderly people in this area.

We conducted a multilevel analysis of the main factors that worsen the eating habits of elderly people. The dependent variable was the food diversity score, and the explanatory variables were living environments (individual attributes, food access, ties with family members and neighbours). We derived the following findings. (1) At the individual level, those who are female, elderly, actively participate in local events and frequently eat with others tend to have healthy eating habits. (2) At the local level, in areas where elderly residents can go outside by themselves and have opportunities to dine with others, residents tend to maintain healthy eating habits. Furthermore, we could find no direct correlation between food access and food diversity scores. This means that weakened ties with family members and neighbours cause unhealthy eating habits among elderly people in the central area of City C.

Then, we classified all neighbourhood associations into groups according to their food diversity scores and living environment factors. The unit of analysis is the neighbourhood associations, of which there are 57 in the city centre. We extracted two types of self-government associations with FDs. These FDs are located in central shopping streets and on the outskirts of the city centre. The former types have good food access, but residents' ties with family members and neighbours (local SC) are extremely weak. The latter type is composed of self-government associations with relatively poor food access and poor ties with family members and neighbours.

Regional City D (Chapter 6)

Regional City D has different areas: urban residential areas for commuters going to Tokyo and agricultural areas where many farmers have lived for many generations. The population of this city was about 85,000 in 2016. We found that most areas without shopping destinations are located in the eastern agricultural areas of this city. However, elderly people at high risk of malnutrition (those with low food diversity scores) live not only in these poor food access agricultural areas but also in the city centres that maintain good food access. Our surveys indicate two main living environment factors that prevent elderly residents from having healthy eating habits: a lack of local SC (weak ties with family members and neighbours) and poor food access (poor shopping environments). These results are different from those of other case studies in central Tokyo and the prefectural governmental city. Poor SC was the most important factor in the occurrence of urban FDs and the influence of food access was limited in these big cities. In contrast, in City D, which is divided into dormitory areas and agricultural areas, not only SC but also food access had a significant influence on elderly peoples' eating habits. It is estimated that SC is important in dormitory towns and food access is important in agricultural areas.

A mobile sales vehicle plays an important role in supporting disadvantaged elderly residents' daily lives in this city. However, the vehicle's stops are mainly around housing complexes. Thus, the sales wagon does not fully cover the residential areas of elderly people at high risk of malnutrition such as poor food access areas in eastern agricultural areas and the weak SC areas in the city centre. In addition, our analyses suggest that patronage of the mobile sales vehicle is high, not only in areas with many elderly people who have difficulty going out on foot (low food access areas), but also in the areas where many elderly people suffer from isolation and poverty (impoverished areas often correspond to low-SC areas). We should assess this shopping support service from the viewpoint of FD issues to improve its effectiveness.

New Food Desert Maps Based on Food Access and Social Capital (Chapter 5)

One of the main purposes of this book is to create new FD maps based on food access and SC. The FD research so far means that food access maps are based on existing statistical data about the locations of people and groceries. However, in urban areas, there is a large gap between the distribution of poor food access areas and that of elderly people at high risk of malnutrition. To develop precise FD maps, we should consider not only food access but also local SC.

In this book, we created a new FD map based on food access and SC in the central areas of a prefectural governmental city. Urban FDs are mainly caused by poor food access and SC. The advantage of this new FD map is that it shows not only FD locations but also the main drivers. If we could extend this map to the whole of Japan, we could implement sustainable and effective countermeasures to overcome FD issues throughout the nation.

However, there are some difficulties in making new FD maps. The first is collecting sufficient individual data from all residents. To measure local SC, we must conduct a large-scale questionnaire survey of all residents of research areas and collect sufficient valid responses. In our research in Chaps. 4–6, owing to the full support of local governments and self-government associations, we collected a sufficient number of valid responses. However, residents do not always co-operate with academic researchers.

The second difficulty is the equivocal nature of the SC measurement index and evaluation criteria (a common index and evaluation criteria are necessary to assess the level of SC in each area). In this book, we chose some SC measurement indices that appear to be suitable measures of elderly people's shopping and eating behaviour. In addition, we identified high or low SC through a comprehensive assessment of our questionnaire responses. However, to establish a common method for FD map creation, we should unify SC measurement indices and clarify the evaluation criteria (if SC falls below the threshold level, isolation from society becomes serious, and has a bad influence on elderly people's eating habits), and these indices and evaluation criteria must be determined based on academic evidence. These are issues to be addressed in the future.

The Introduction of Noteworthy Countermeasures Against Food Deserts (Chapter 7)

In Chap. 7, we introduced countermeasures against FDs. Many countermeasures have been implemented throughout the entire nation and can be classified into three types: dining together, food delivery, and improving food access. Appropriate services are provided by diverse actors, such as local people, municipalities, and private companies.

The problems these countermeasures encounter are their low profitability and low sustainability. Many providers of countermeasure services have gone bankrupt owing to the shortcomings of their operations. On the other hand, some pioneering organizations have developed elaborate business models to ensure business sustainability. Their business models can be classified as follows: business expansion; entry from a different industry; co-operation with different industries; resident volunteering; co-operation with industry, government, schools, and local community; welfare businesses; and new businesses.

Future Countermeasures Against Urban Food Deserts

We would like to point out the following four findings based on the knowledge gained from our research in this book.

The Necessity of Paying Attention to Urban Areas

The present countermeasures mainly apply in poor food access areas, including agricultural regions, mountain villages, fishing villages, and old housing complexes. However, as we mentioned in this book, the most serious FDs occur in urban areas. In addition, the elderly population will increase rapidly in urban areas in the near future. From the viewpoint of preventive care, especially for senior citizens, we should attend to urban areas and develop their living environments. It is safe to say that the most important living environment factor is local SC. We must put more emphasis on 'How do we supply hot meals to isolated elderly people?' rather than 'How do w e deliver food systematically to elderly people in poor food access areas?'.

Share a Common Recognition That Food Desert Countermeasures Are Unprofitable and Improve Their Sustainability

In the early 2000s, when the expression 'Kaimono Jakusya' (disadvantaged shopper) became popular, the mass media often proclaimed that Kaimono Jakusya would become a new big business opportunity, and many people believed them. Many new countermeasures such as mobile sales wagons and roundsman services started throughout the nation. However, at the present time, many have gone bankrupt and ceased operations. Food desert countermeasures are not profitable businesses.

The authors are researchers and we have no experience of retailing or social welfare services. However, we have researched many kinds of countermeasures. In addition, we are members of boards commissioned with applying national government countermeasures and some local government countermeasures. From these experiences, we realize how difficult it is to manage sustainable countermeasures to FD issues.[3] Enthusiasm is important to support elderly people, but it is insufficient to sustain these support services. To achieve sustainable support, not only passionate enthusiasm but also careful and profitable business plans are necessary. In our experience, many applicants for government subsidies to address FD issues have great enthusiasm but lack thorough business plans and judgement. Business plans that rely entirely on subsidies are difficult to sustain.

However, the pioneer countermeasures we introduced in this book can maintain their profitability in many ways. These cases offer many suggestions for business operators seeking to establish sustainable business models. In addition, in economics and distribution science, there are many discussions about obtaining profit from FD countermeasures (Jimyong 2015; Kiuchi 2015).

We must accept the premise that FD countermeasures are not profitable. Then, we should discuss how to create new business models to operate sustainable and profitable countermeasures against FDs.

Methods of Supplying Fresh Food (Co-operation with Local Residents, Private Companies, and Local Governments to Promote Healthy Dietary Education)

Previous FD studies have considered how to improve food delivery systems in poor food access areas. However, in urban FDs, the most serious problem is how to deliver hot meals to isolated elderly people rather than how to deliver food to elderly people in poor food access areas. We would like to mention the following two important points.

First, food supply systems operate in co-operation with local people. Many elderly people live in urban FDs, isolated from families and local society, and have little will to maintain healthy eating habits. For these people, nearby grocery shops to which they are not accustomed are distant in their minds. If the staff members of these faraway shops recommend that elderly people purchase healthy food, isolated elderly people are hardly likely to follow their advice. As we mentioned in Chap. 7, people tend to follow advice from key local people (such as leaders of the local community, welfare commissioners, and charity workers). If these key local people advise elderly people to change their eating habits, they often purchase healthy foods and eat them. It may be that these local people can improve isolated elderly people's lifestyles. On the other hand, to provide a stable supply of safe and healthy foods to carless elderly people, support from retailing companies is necessary. Furthermore, local governments can establish effective collaborations between local people and retailers. Therefore, co-operation between local residents, private companies, and local governments is important in establishing sustainable and effective FD countermeasures.

The second point is healthy diet education. Many elderly people seem to lack awareness of healthy eating habits. In our questionnaire surveys of central Tokyo (Chap. 4) and the prefectural governmental city (Chap. 5), many residents reported that 'I eat healthy meals every day'. However, the food diversity survey showed that almost half of them actually have poor eating habits and are at high risk of malnutrition. This suggests that many residents lack awareness of healthy eating habits. To improve their dietary habits, the promotion of healthy diet education is necessary.[4] Healthy diet education is also important for middle-aged people approaching old age. It is very hard for elderly people to change their lifestyles. If people learn healthy eating and cooking skills while they are young, it is expected that they will practise better habits in their later years.

Sharing of the Database by Industry, Government, and Universities

To operate sustainable and effective countermeasures, we must clarify who needs support, where they live, and what kind of support they need. The types of elderly people who need support have changed rapidly in a short period of time. For example, in the case of the mobile sales wagon, the main users are elderly people who support themselves enough to cook, but seldom go shopping at distant grocery shops by themselves. However, if their health deteriorates as they age, cooking and shopping will become difficult. Then, their needs will change from the mobile sales wagon service to a nursing care service. On the other hand, it becomes more difficult with age to go shopping. Therefore, the number of elderly people who need shopping support is continuously increasing, and the disadvantaged shoppers are distributed randomly. Therefore, it is very difficult for retailers through their own efforts to keep collecting information about where disadvantaged shoppers live.

The senior citizens' welfare divisions of city councils usually keep detailed raw data about elderly people's personal situations and their living environments. However, because these data are personally identifiable, there are strict restrictions on who can see them. Thus, researchers seldom analyse these raw data directly. I f governments delete personally identifiable information from these raw data and make a database that researchers can access, interdisciplinary researchers will analyse it and offer useful findings. For example, if we analyse the database, we can make new FD maps like those described in Chap. 5 on a national scale.[5] By employing the useful information offered by researchers, operational bodies could develop more beneficial and sustainable FD countermeasures.

Future FD Problems (FD in New Lifestyles After the New Corona Virus Pandemic)

The FD issues in Japan, Europe, and the USA are similar in terms of the health damage to residents attributable to the worsening of their shopping environment and the deterioration of eating habits. However, we can see some differences. The largest difference between Japanese FDs and those in Europe and the USA is the characteristics of victims. In Europe and the USA, the main victims of FD issues are low-income households such as foreign unskilled labourers and single mothers. In contrast, in Japan, isolated elderly people with little support from families and neighbours are most seriously affected. Europe and the USA have seriously widening social gaps, and poverty is the basis of FD issues. However, weakened ties with family members and neighbours (weakened SC) are the basis of Japanese FD issues.

Japan and other east Asian countries are similar in many aspects. There have been few FD studies in East Asian countries except for Japan. However, many background factors of Japanese FDs are common to other east Asian countries. Declining birth rates and a growing proportion of elderly people are not uniquely Japanese problems. For example, the total fertility rate in 2018 was quite low in east Asian countries: Korea (1.0), Taiwan (1.1), Japan (1.42), and China (1.7) (United Nations 2019).

Traditionally, Asian people have lived with large families and maintained good relationships with neighbours. Therefore, family members or neighbours generally support socially vulnerable people such as the elderly (see Segawa 2004). However, as we mentioned in Chaps. 2 and 3, a declining birth rate, a growing proportion of elderly people, and changes of lifestyle caused by economic growth often weaken ties with family members and neighbours. We can see these phenomena not only in Japan but also in other Asian countries. These changes often cause Japanese-type FD issues.

Therefore, in the near future, Japanese-type FD issues will arise in many Asian countries (or already have). Some European countries also have strong family ties and suffer from declining birth rates and a growing elderly population. Therefore, these countries possibly have FD issues similar to those in Japan.

Japan used to be a society of low economic disparities. However, the proportion of people living in relative poverty has recently increased. The proportion of people in relative poverty was 12.0% in 1985, but it reached 15.7% in 2015 (Ministry of Health, Labour and Welfare: MHLW 2017). About half of these poor households are single-parent families. Hence, poverty is a serious problem among children of low-income households. In addition, the number of foreign workers is increasing, reaching about 1.66 million in 2019 (MHLW 2020). Therefore, we are afraid that European and US-type FDs may arise in Japan in the near future.

Three years have passed since we published this book in Japanese in 2017. During these three years, unfortunately, we have observed few positive changes in relation to FD issues in Japan (as of August 2020). On the other hand, the new coronavirus pandemic must be considered the most significant negative change since 2017. We can find little sign of the end of the pandemic at present. New lifestyles (the 'new normal') after the pandemic, such as maintaining social distance and using business-to-business e-commerce will have a substantial influence on our lives. In the case of shopping, expanding online ordering and delivery services may develop the living environments of shopping-disadvantaged people in poor food access areas. In fact, some countermeasures such as healthy ready-meal delivery and mobile vending vehicle increase their sales (i.e. Chap. 7, Sects. 7.2.4 and 7.2.5). However, as we pointed out in this book, the essentials of Japanese FD issues are isolation from society (low SC) and poverty. The coronavirus pandemic must make these issues more serious from now on. As we mentioned in Chap. 7, some innovative countermeasures have begun in Japan (i.e. Chap. 7, Sects. 7.2.3, 7.2.4, and 7.2.7). Although many remain unprofitable, they offer good suggestions for tackling FD issues.

Measurement of FD issues corresponds to some of the Sustainable Development Goals, such as 'good health and well-being', 'reducing inequality', and 'sustainable cities and communities'. In addition, the importance of studying and tackling FD issues is likely to increase in the future. Japanese FD studies may be useful in other Asian countries, and previous European and US studies may be useful in Japan. We should share information about FD issues and discuss them together more.

Notes

1. The distance between a home and a nearby grocery shop.
2. We published the Japanese version of this book in 2017 (Iwama 2017). This book is a revised English version.
3. In the distribution and economic science fields, many researchers point out the difficulty of gaining sufficient profit from FD countermeasures (Asakawa and Kato 2012; Jimyong 2013).
4. Even in poor food access areas, many elderly people mainly purchase lunch boxes, snacks, and convenience foods from mobile sales wagons. This shows the necessity of healthy diet education.
5. As we mentioned in Chap. 3, the Japan Agency for Gerontological Evaluation Study (JAGES) project was a pioneer case (JAGES HP: http://www.jages.net/).

References

Asakawa Y, Kato T (2012) The business of supporting 'shopping refugees' and its profitability. Manage Res 63(3):19–38 (Japanese)

Iwama N (ed) (2011) Japanese food deserts. Association of Agriculture and Forestry Statistics, Tokyo (Japanese)

Iwama N (ed) (2017) Japanese Urban food deserts. Association of Agriculture and Forestry Statistics, Tokyo (Japanese)

Jimyong L (2013) A study on the mission of logistics and its measures for the aged society. J Univ Mark Distrib Sci. Distribution sciences & business administration 26:69–86

Jimyong L (2015) Study on the business model of rolling stores for restricted shoppers. J Univ Mark Distrib Sci 28:27–40

Kikuchi H (2015) Food deserts and retail sale management. J Bus Adm 85:111–127 (Japanese)

Ministry of Health, Labour and Welfare (2017) Annual report on health, labor and welfare: social security and economic growth (Japanese). https://www.mhlw.go.jp/wp/hakusyo/kousei/17/index.html. Accessed 14 Aug 2020

Ministry of Health, Labour and Welfare (2020) The notification status of foreign workers' employment status (as of end October 2020) (Japanese). https://www.mhlw.go.jp/stf/newpage_09109.html. Accessed 14 Aug 2020

Segawa M (2004) Anthropology of Chinese society: from relatives and families. Sekaishiso seminar, Kyoto (Japanese)

United Nations: Department of Economic and Social Affairs Population Dynamics (2019) World Population Prospects 2019. https://population.un.org/wpp/. Accessed 14 Aug 2020